ON the Go
Tales of a Trauma Flight Nurse

GREG McCAFFREY,
RN, MICN, MICP

Copyright © 2019 Greg McCaffrey, RN, MICN, MICP
All rights reserved
First Edition

PAGE PUBLISHING, INC.
New York, NY

First originally published by Page Publishing, Inc. 2019

ISBN 978-1-64462-792-1 (Paperback)
ISBN 978-1-64462-794-5 (Hardcover)
ISBN 978-1-64462-793-8 (Digital)

Printed in the United States of America

To the men and women of Emergency Services.

My first book, On the Go

CONTENTS

1 The Bridge 7
2 First Call...23
3 Highway 50 36
4 Feather River Plane Crash....................................46
5 Long Night in Bi-County 72
6 Wrong Way, Tony 101
7 Chester Snowmobile 113
8 Scotty's 123
9 Charcoal and Ewald 131
10 Drive-Ups...139
11 911 Follies..144
12 The New Recruit..148
13 Mom and Baby...159
14 Highway 70 Rescue 175
15 Horsing Around 186
16 Idle Time..199
17 A Valuable Lesson...216
18 Fountain Fire..228
19 Medical Legal 242
20 Trip to Sacramento 253
21 Home at Last..271

1

THE BRIDGE

"**OKAY, YOU GUYS**, sit down and buckle up!" I demand as I'm looking over my shoulder into the back seat of our quad cab Dodge Ram. As I turn back around, my son Colby just looks at me in the mirror with a "Really?" look on his face. I just smile back, start up the engine, and put it into gear. Colby and three of his teammates are riding with me as an entire convoy of cars, trucks, and minivans pulls away from the Portola High School and starts the long trip down the Feather River Canyon to a basketball game in Maxwell. As a parent, we are expected to help out with the transportation of the kids during the high school basketball season. In reality, I really enjoy it. The boys are a good group of kids, and the conversation is fun.

My number one rule if you're traveling in my truck is, you can't wear a headset to listen to music. The first time I took the boys, I suddenly realized how quiet it was and looked around to see that all of them were wearing headsets, listening to iPods. I immediately pulled the truck over and demanded they take them off. I then told them, if they wanted to listen to music, give one of the iPods to me and I'd plug it into the truck's stereo. With questioning and scared looks on their faces, they coughed up one of the iPods and we plugged it in. Instantly, Colby wanted to know why they couldn't listen to their own music. I replied by telling him that they should engage into some good, old-fashioned conversation. All their eyes rolled at that time. He then asked what they were supposed to talk about, and I answered, "Something will come up." Before long, all the boys were actively engaged into a conversation. At first, yes, it was about me and what a hard-ass I was being, but I got my point across and soon they were all joking around and didn't stop talking and laughing until I pulled into the McDonald's in Oroville two hours later. As they jumped out of the truck to get their Big Macs, fries, and chocolate shakes, I walked in grinning, knowing I had proved my point.

Some of the other parents have also arrived, and we are all trying to figure out how much farther the ride will be, and also with the understanding that we will not be back home until around one or two in the morning, we know it is going be a long night.

As we load back up in the truck, all the boys are laughing and kidding around, and I start out of the parking lot, heading west on state Route 162 when I notice that we are about to cross the Feather River over the new bridge. This project was just being proposed when I left the area ten years ago. I can also see the old metal bridge just off to the north. It appears to have been saved as a footbridge for joggers and bicyclists. As we are starting onto the new bridge, I notice a dedication sign, and as I strain to read it in passing, I am suddenly speechless and feel cold chills running down my back. Colby notices my change in behavior and asks, "What's up?"

I only tell him, "Nothing. Something I ate."

During the remaining trip to Maxwell, the boys are all talking and laughing, but I'm not hearing them. I can't get the name of the bridge out of my mind.

We stay for all four of the games at Maxwell, and it doesn't take long after we load back up and take off, headed for home, that all the boys are completely passed out and I'm not going to have to stop again until we reach Portola.

It is about eleven o'clock at night when I am rolling back into Oroville and slowing as I approach the bridge once again. This time, as I cross, I want to read the sign to make sure what I read earlier was in fact whom this bridge was dedicated to.

I slow the truck, and as I reach the sign at the beginning of the bridge, I bump the headlights up to high beam. I'm almost stopped in the road as I read, "Randy Jennings Memorial Bridge." I read it several times before I take my foot off the brake and step on the accelerator once again.

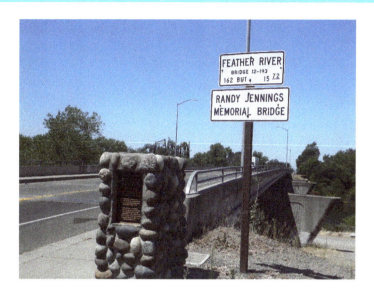

As I pull onto the freeway and head north on Highway 70 into the dark, moonless night, memories of a tragic night start to fill my consciousness.

I start to recall my time working in Chico at Enloe Medical Center, the helicopter, ambulances, and working in the emergency department. One of the things the emergency department and FlightCare staff could do is to sign up for on-call shifts, hoping we would be called in. The overtime is great, and out-of-town transfers could be a fun thing to do on your day off to make extra money. Such was this day, May 21, 1997, a day I will never forget.

I have been called in to take a transfer from Chico to the University of California–Stanford in Palo Alto. The trip down there is about five to six hours. After you transfer care of the patient over to the nurses and physicians, the rest of the trip is pretty much open to do what you would like to do. We have to drive through San Francisco on the way home, and of course, we have to stop at Fisherman's Wharf to have clam chowder for lunch and load up on San Francisco french bread to take home. All in all, there really is no hurry to get home. Since this is an overtime shift, we simply turn in our paperwork and go home. The entire round trip usually runs about eleven to twelve hours.

THE BRIDGE

After filling our stomachs with great food, we leave San Francisco and the Bay Area and eventually jump off Interstate 80 onto Interstate 5 and head north. Eventually, we will leave I-5 and head across the back roads. As we are getting closer to our home in Butte County, we start picking up radio traffic in the area and commenting on what a nice evening it is.

In Oroville, Randy, a Butte County Sheriff deputy, is just waking prior to his night shift. He knows tomorrow is his wife's birthday, and he wants to surprise her this evening with her present. Terry has been trying to be quiet around the house during the day, knowing he needs his sleep, but at the same time, she is getting ready for a birthday dinner in Chico with some of her friends from the Oroville Police Department. As the two of them sit and discuss some of the events of the day and their previous shifts with the different law enforcement agencies, they both feel their lives are totally on track and couldn't be better.

Randy has just been accepted into the County SWAT team, something he has been working toward for some time, and Terry has started her new dog with the Oroville PD's K-9 unit.

After downing a Gatorade, Randy can't take the suspense any longer and takes Terry out to her truck, otherwise known to the two of them as the dog car. He wants to show her the new stereo he has installed. He has also sneaked out and has it all set up and already turned on. As Terry approaches, she can't help but notice it is playing Pachelbel's Canon in D, her favorite, and she sits in the truck, smiling and listening before giving him a big hug and kiss for all his effort.

Randy looks at his watch and knows he has to get ready for work and, leaving Terry in the truck, heads back into the house to shower and get dressed into his uniform.

Terry is also getting ready for her evening with her friends, and the two of them meet one last time prior to heading out in their own directions. Terry can't help but notice how handsome he looks in his uniform, and Randy does the same, looking at Terry all made up for a night out with the girls. A last kiss followed by Randy telling her to have fun, and Terry also telling him to be careful.

Randy then heads out in his patrol car, and Terry jumps into her truck and heads out to Chico, listening to music on her new stereo. She meets up with her friends and, over the next hour, has a great time. She will be forty tomorrow, and everyone wants to comment on that. *I guess you can't be twenty-nine forever,* she thinks.

Randy is patrolling in town with a huge smile on his face. He knows the present he has gotten for Terry is perfect and she will enjoy it for years; he isn't even really thinking much about searching out for bad guys, as he knows this is Oroville, and so they will make themselves known.

It is a little before ten o'clock when Randy hears two deputies responding to a domestic violence call and, shortly after, hears a report that the assailant, an Oriental man, has fled the scene and is last seen running south toward Grant Avenue and possibly has a gun. About the same time, a report comes in from a CHP officer in the area of someone fitting that description running into a grassy field behind a church. Randy knows he is probably the closest to that area and calls in that he will head to that location.

He arrives at the church and sees a man fitting the description running into the field next to the church. He yells for the suspect to stop, then loses sight of him in the tall grass. Just then, the sergeant that has been at the suspect's home arrives, and Randy starts running through the field to the location he has last seen the suspect, and the sergeant does the same, following about fifty feet behind him.

Our conversation in the ambulance comes to a halt when we hear the sheriff dispatch channel coming alive with the pursuit. We listen intently as the two deputies have been dispatched to a man with a gun in an area of Oroville well-known to me as a bad area of town. As we turn down the volume on our conversation and turn up the volume on the radio, we hear that there are now two deputies in foot pursuit of a suspect with a gun. As our attention is now totally focused, I start to think what the Oroville ambulance personnel will be thinking and what may happen if one of the deputies ends up shooting the suspect.

Terry has finished her dinner with her friends and is enjoying her thirty-minute ride back to Oroville. She is smiling, listening to her new stereo, thinking about Randy and how nice it is of him to not only get her a new stereo but also have it installed and ready for her this evening. As she is entering Oroville, she sees a sheriff car speeding through town, lights and sirens flashing and wailing, and thinks to herself, *Someone is having a bad night.*

Randy is running through the field, gun drawn, and the sergeant is trying to catch up when suddenly, a man jumps up from the three-foot-tall grass and, without warning, starts firing. Randy and the sergeant are surprised by the flashes of light coming from the barrel of the suspect's gun. Randy doesn't even think; his instincts and training have kicked in, and before he even thinks about it, his gun is in front of him and he is returning fire. The sergeant has stopped as he hears the banging of both guns firing in front of him and the whistling of bullets passing all around him, but because he is directly behind Randy, he can't return fire.

Just as sudden as the shooting has started, it stops. The sergeant, holding his gun in front of him, keys up the radio and, with adrenaline pumping, announces over the radio, "SHOTS FIRED, SHOTS FIRED!"

Looking at my partner in the ambulance, I say, "Well, I guess that answers that," thinking the armed suspect is now entering the trauma system or, possibly, the morgue. Our thoughts are suddenly stunned with the next transmission.

Randy has dropped to one knee, knowing he has taken several rounds from the suspect's gun, but not knowing if they have all been taken in his Kevlar vest or into other parts of his body or how bad things actually may be. He grabs the microphone, keys the transmit button, and in a surprisingly calm voice, announces to Butte County, "I'm hit. Send an ambulance!" Then he collapses to the ground.

My partner and I look, staring at each other, not wanting to say anything but wanting to ask, "Do you think a deputy has been hit?" Before we can even open up the conversation, the radio comes back to life when the sergeant has knelt down next to Randy, quickly assessing the situation, and calls over the radio to dispatch, "OFFICER DOWN, OFFICER DOWN! SEND THE MEDICS!"

Unbelievable is all I can think as I now can hear the tones for the Oroville ambulance. "Wow, that doesn't sound good," I say to my partner. As we travel the back roads across the valley, getting closer to Chico, we enter into some conversation about different shootings we have seen in our careers and some of the different circumstances surrounding them.

Within a few minutes, we hear the Oroville ambulance arrive on the scene and, within seconds, radio back to their base, "Dispatch, the helicopter, immediately!" As we now hear the tones sounding for the flight crew, I can tell my partner has pushed a little harder on the throttle. I don't blame him; I would like to get back to the hospital to see what is going on myself. We both know, if we have this planned out correctly, we should be getting back to Chico just as the helicopter is returning from Oroville and landing at Enloe.

In the distance, we can see the lights of Chico and have been able to pick out the flashing lights of the helicopter as it makes its way south toward Oroville, which is only a quick fifteen-minute flight. As we enter the Chico city limits, we hear the helicopter calling in that they are now en route back and requesting a trauma team activation with an ETA of ten minutes. They follow this with their radio report.

"Enloe Dispatch, FlightCare, ten-minute ETA. On board we have a thirty-eight-year-old male deputy sheriff with multiple gunshot wounds. One to his left arm and one to his anterior chest just below his left clavicle and lateral to the sternum. Currently, his level of consciousness is decreasing. He is only moaning to pain. Vital signs are, blood pressure 76 over 40, heart rate 150, and respirations 26. Two IVs established and running, and oxygen per nonrebreather mask at 15 liters per minute."

The driver and I both look at each other and don't say a word. We don't have to. This doesn't sound good. As we pull up onto the ambulance dock at Enloe, we hear the helicopter radio in with an update, and there is obvious excitement in the nurse's voice. "CPR in progress!" Nothing more needs to be said.

As Terry arrives back at her house, she is still excited about the dinner she has just had with her friends and decides to call another one of her friends at the Oroville Police Dispatch Center, knowing she is getting off shift soon, and wants to see if she wants to go for a walk with her after work. When her friend answers the phone and an upbeat Terry asks about the walk, there is a pause, as if her friend is at a loss for words. She then asks if the sergeant has been to her house. Instantly suspicious, Terry tells her no, then notices headlights pulling up at the front gate. She tells her friend a car is just pulling up and she will call her back in a few minutes, then starts out to the gate to find Sergeant Keeler and a lieutenant and jokingly says, "I don't know if I should ask for representation or offer snacks!" But then she notices the seriousness of their faces as Sergeant Keeler walks up to her and tells her, "Randy has been shot! He is on his way to Enloe in Chico."

Stunned, now feeling as if her breath has been sucked from her lungs, she finds it hard to breathe as the sergeant gently reaches out to her. Defensively, Terry shakes the grasp from her arm and is now not hearing any words from either of the officers. She jumps into her truck and, with the throttle floored, races past the two and leaves them in a cloud of dust. She suddenly thinks of her mother-in-law and, grabbing the cell phone, tries to call her but finds the battery is dead. Within a few minutes, she comes to a screeching halt at her mother-in-law's house and starts banging on the door and windows, yelling out for her to wake up.

A light comes on in the house, and Terry is met at the front door by Randy's mother with a surprised look on her face. Terry doesn't give her a chance to speak, just telling her, "Randy has been shot! Grab your purse. We need to go!"

As the two of them leave the Oroville city limits, Terry is suddenly frustrated with the governor of her truck that won't let her drive any faster than one hundred miles per hour. The ride to Chico seems to take hours. During the ride, she is faced with a plethora of thoughts and emotions flooding her mind. *How bad is he wounded? Will he be crippled? Can he walk?* The list just keeps growing as it seems that she is just creeping along, minute after slow minute, mile after slow mile.

The two of them pull up to the main entrance of the hospital. They run into the waiting room and tell the receptionist, "My husband has been brought here. He has been shot." The receptionist asks the women to wait where they are and she will go get someone to help them. Not wanting to wait, and Randy's mother being a vocational nurse for many years and knowing her way around a hospital, the two take the matter into their own hands and decide to go into the emergency department and search room by room, bed by bed, until they find him.

As I step out of the ambulance at the hospital, I can hear the beating of the helicopter blades as it is making its landing above me on the helipad, and I am already thinking to myself as I enter through the electric doors all the different things the trauma team will be tasked into doing and that, more than likely, they will be opening up the deputy's chest as soon as he enters the trauma room.

The trauma room is the first room on the left as you enter the hallway. Located near the ambulance dock, it saves a lot of time not having to wind your way down hallways with critical patients. As I approach the door to the room, I take a peek in and can see the trauma team already assembled and wearing their gowns and x-ray aprons. Looking around, I spot Drena standing in the corner, and I send her a wave. As I'm turning to continue down the hall and put my paperwork away and grab my truck keys, I suddenly hear the nurse from the trauma room yelling out, "Hey, Greg, can you come in here and help me?" *Crap, I shouldn't have stuck my head in.* Before I can say anything, I can hear him asking the charge nurse if it is okay if I stay and help. "Yes," she says, without asking me any questions or if I wouldn't mind, and definitely without thinking I have already been working twelve hours. She points to the room and says, "Go help him, please."

"Okay," I answer back as I turn to walk down the hall to the locker room and set down my gear, but I am stopped when I spot the flight crew approaching. One of them is ventilating the patient, while the other is squeezing IV bags and the ED tech has his feet on the side rail of the gurney, riding it as he is performing chest compressions. I quickly set my stuff down on the nurse's station desk and run into the room to grab an x-ray apron. I can see that Drena has heard our conversation, and she is standing there with an x-ray gown open for me. I thrust my arms through the openings and turn around almost in one movement. She then quickly ties the nylon straps in the back for me as I pull on a pair of gloves, and just as I snap the second glove on, the patient and flight crew enter the room.

The first thing I notice is the deputy's uniform. His shirt has been cut up the middle, and parts of his duty belt are hanging off both sides of the gurney. I see the stripe running down the side of his pants and his black boots. A quick look back up, and I see his chest is covered in blood, and every time the ED tech pushes down for a chest compression, blood squirts out of a bullet hole in his chest. The tech is having a difficult time keeping his latex-gloved hands in place, as they are covered in blood and sliding with each of the compressions. He also has blood splatter on his face and running down his shirt from the blood spurting out of the wound.

As we are moving the deputy over to the ED gurney, the flight crew is giving a loud verbal report, which the trauma nurse is trying to write down on some scratch paper, which she will transcribe onto the trauma form later. The trauma surgeon doesn't seem to be listening, as he has his stethoscope in his ears, holding the diaphragm on the deputy's chest, trying to listen for heart sounds.

The flight nurse hasn't finished her report when the surgeon stands back and, in a soft but matter-of-fact voice, looks at me and says, "Hand me a scalpel!" I don't need any further explanation. I know he is going to open the deputy's chest, and rightfully so. The deputy has been bleeding out into his chest all the way from Oroville. There is no need for x-rays, lab, urine samples; this guy needs his chest opened to find what is bleeding and fix it, now!

The trauma nurse has already pulled the chest thoracotomy tray out, and I quickly pull open the last sterile fold that is covering it, exposing all the equipment. I roll the tray over to the surgeon, and he pulls the scalpel from the kit. As he is feeling for the landmarks, trying to identify where to start his incision, I quickly grab the Betadine spray bottle and spray the deputy's chest, including the surgeon's hands. Without hesitation, he starts making an incision around the deputy's left chest through the skin, running just above a rib. The deputy is a large man, and the incision runs from his scapula all the way around his side to his sternum. After he finishes the first incision, he retraces it now with a deeper incision all the way into the chest. The surgeon pushes his finger into the chest and will now use his finger as a guide inside the chest as he makes the final full-depth incision along the same wound. The finger inside will make sure that he won't be cutting any internal organs.

As he starts this second incision, I am standing directly beside him and watching as a small amount of blood starts out, then as the incision grows, larger amounts of blood start out of the chest. When he reaches about ten inches, a massive amount of blood dumps out of the chest, hitting the floor and splattering all over anything within five feet of the gurney. I can now feel the warm blood running down my legs as I am directly in front of the spill, and behind me I hear the trauma nurse voice an, "Oh, shit!" as she watches what looks like a couple liters of blood covering everyone and now running down the wall and cabinets at the head of the bed.

The surgeon has finished his incision, and I have grabbed the rib spreaders off the chest tray. I hold them out for him, and without looking away from his incision, he tells the ED tech to stop chest compressions and asks the two of us to open the chest so he can look inside. I take a quick look up at the tech and know we have been in this position before. He is already on the right side of the gurney, and I'm on the left. We both work our fingers into the incision, and as we both start pulling the chest apart, the surgeon keeps cutting to let the chest open wider. As he is doing this, more blood is hitting the floor, and I can feel my feet starting to slip on the blood-soaked floor. Looking up, I spot the fight paramedic and yell for him to grab the suction from the wall-mounted unit. The surgeon is now trying to look into the chest and, at first, inspects the heart to see if it is wounded or has a tamponade. The paramedic hands me the suction, and with my free hand, I stick it into the chest to try to suction some of the blood that is flowing from some unknown wound. I run the tip of the suction around the heart, then further into the chest between the wall and the lung, trying to open a pathway for the surgeon to explore, looking for the cause of the bleeding.

The other ED nurse has been trying to direct one of the large overhead lights into the wound, but because of the surgeon and the two of us holding the chest apart, she just can't get the right angle. So finally giving up, she grabs a smaller suture light that is on wheels—

but it is still very bright—and somehow wiggles it up between us and is able to shine it into the open chest.

The surgeon is trying so hard to find the wound and finally realizes he does not have enough hands. He grabs the suction from me and then tells me to reach in and hold the patient's heart and lung out of the way. I place one hand into the open chest, gently pushing the heart aside, then start pushing the lung aside, and as I do this, I can see and feel the lung expanding and contracting as each breath of oxygen is being squeezed into him by the respiratory therapist. Now looking in, I can see where the surgeon is trying to get, and I'm able to help move the heart and lung the best I can to clear a path for him as he works his way first toward the center of the chest, then up toward the top of the rib cage, following the aorta.

Finally, I notice him pausing. His head is now only inches from the large opening as he struggles to look deep into the chest, then readjusting the light and feeling inside along the great vessels, he says, "I found it!" We all hold our breath, waiting for him to tell us what to do next.

Time, which is flashing past us now, seems to be standing still, as if the second hand on the clock has suddenly stopped. He studies the wound for a few more seconds as we all hold our breath, then looking up at the ED tech and me, he says, "The bullet has torn his left subclavian artery completely off the aorta. The whole area is destroyed."

We continue to look at the surgeon as he stands up, turns his head, and looks at the flat line on the cardiac monitor, asking, "Does he have a heartbeat?" We already know that answer, and now looking back down at Randy's heart, which is my hand, I can see that it is not beating, not even quivering, and has turned blue. The surgeon then takes a step back, looking at the deputy, then the monitors once again, and asks the recording nurse, "What time is it?"

We know what this means; he wants to know the time so he can document what time he is pronouncing him. "It's twenty-three zero six," she replies. There is a pause in all the people in the room. Not a word is spoken. Silence. Finally, the surgeon speaks up, "That's it, he's gone!"

The ED tech and I slowly pull our hands out of the deputy's chest. As we both take a step back and straighten our backs, it is the first time I have really had a chance to take in the entire room. I slowly scan the area and see that most the faces of all the members of the trauma team are welling up with tears. We know this was one of the good guys. We don't understand all the circumstances of the evening but do know that it is people like this that make our world, the world we live in, a better and safer place. We've all worked so hard, and the members of the team, x-ray, lab, and the OR nurses, that really didn't get to do their part feel as if they didn't get to help. There is a feeling of helplessness to all of us. My eyes finally stop when I spot Drena standing in the back of the room. She is staring at me, and from across the room, I can see she is fighting back tears from running down her face.

I want to walk over and give her a hug, to wipe her tears, but then I take a look at myself and can see that I'm covered in blood. It is still running down my arms and the yellow x-ray apron, dripping onto the floor, and I can feel its warmth on the front of my legs, as it has soaked through my pants. Also, what I thought were beads of sweet running down my face are actually more blood splatters. I look at the ED tech and the surgeon, and they have not fared any better. We are all still in a trance, pulling our thoughts together, trying to shift gears and come up with a plan as to what to do next, when we are all interrupted by two people bursting into the room.

In shock, we look up and see two women. A quick look, and I recognize Terry from my shifts working in Oroville. A shiver goes down my spine as I realize she is Randy's wife. At the same time, I notice others in the room I hadn't noticed before. Some are dressed in uniforms, some plain clothes. I can only guess they are all deputies or police officers.

Terry is now staring at the lifeless body on the gurney. His arms are draped off to the side, hands blue, chest still wide-open, blood dripping from all of us, running down the wall and cabinets. The floor is covered in blood with footprints and smudges where we have been slipping and sliding, which are still fresh and glistening. Taking all this in, she grabs her face and lets out a scream. Those in the room that weren't crying are now horrified and are trying to get out, away from this scene.

As Terry slowly walks up to her husband's side, I grab a sheet from the shelf, and the ED tech and I rapidly try to cover up Randy's chest. I know I can't clean the room as it is now a crime scene, and the investigators from the sheriff's office will be coming to slowly remove and log into evidence each item from the deputy. As I step away, I see that someone has removed some of the items that have either fallen off his uniform or have been removed and set them on the counter next to the sink. I didn't notice until now, but the county sheriff has also responded and is in the room as well. He and Terry are now having some words as she is voicing her frustration, and the sheriff is letting her. He has lost a deputy, but she has lost a husband. As I stand at the sink and start to clean some of the blood from my face and arms, I notice Drena has walked up alongside me and, without saying a word, simply leans against me. Soon she asks if she can do anything. I ask her if she could try to find me some scrubs so I can change. After giving me a second gentle nudge, she walks out of the room.

As I am cleaning myself, I notice the items on the counter, and lying under some items, I spot the deputy's badge. It is covered in blood. I don't know how it got off his uniform or over to the counter but, I'm very appreciative that it didn't get lost. I know I am not supposed to do this, but at this point, I don't care. I take the badge and rinse it off in the flowing water in the sink. As I pull some paper towels to dry the badge and my hands, I turn to look the scene over. Terry has stepped away from her husband for a moment, and I take the opportunity to walk over and place the badge on the white-and-red bloody sheet that is covering Randy's chest.

Soon, Drena has returned with some scrubs, and I take the opportunity while waiting for Terry to spend some time with her husband to run to the nurse's lounge and take a quick shower and change into the scrubs. After what seems like an hour, I return to the trauma room just as Terry is leaving, and I choke up, watching her being helped out of the hospital. I have never been able to handle the family dynamics that cases like this produce.

ON THE GO

As Terry and her mother-in-law start their trip back to Oroville, she is having trouble seeing the road, with tears streaming from her face when she notices a song on the radio, the radio Randy has just had installed for her. The song is Trisha Yearwood's "How Do I Live without You."

I enter the room and find two deputies from the sheriff department that have been requested to take over the investigation. I check in with the deputies and ask if they need anything. They tell me that they don't think so, as they usually bring all their own equipment, but will ask if needed. I then tell them that this is still an active ER and there will be hospital staff in and out of the room, gathering equipment. They don't like it but also know that there is no option. We agree to help keep the traffic to a minimum and not disturb them. I then ask if I can start cleaning up some of the room, pointing to the blood running off the walls and cabinets, knowing that the longer it is there, the harder it is to get off. They look around and can see that the room is a mess and agree, only after they photograph everything. Agreed, I walk back to the cleaning room and grab a mop bucket and an armful of towels. As I set them down in the room, the deputy finishes with the room pictures and gives me the go-ahead to start cleaning.

As I start literally mopping down the walls, I can't help but listen to the two deputies systematically removing, photographing, documenting, and placing each and every item into paper bags that are then marked with the case number. Eventually, I enter into a conversation with them as they get closer to finishing with the task at hand and are just making sure they have everything they think they will need. I ask about the shooter and if they have any information on him. Not fully aware of the details of the scene, they fill me in that Randy had indeed shot the man he was chasing in what was described as an incredible shootout and they understand that he was pronounced dead at the scene.

As the two deputies finish, the mortician and his wife arrive. Terry has called them as they are very dear friends of both her and Randy, and with the help of the ED tech, we gently move Randy onto the mortician's gurney and help him close the body bag. I help push the gurney out onto the ambulance dock, and after we load it into the back of the mortician's van, his wife steps up and climbs into the back, unzips the body bag, and tells us that she wants to ride in the back and hold Randy's hand on his final trip home.

As I walk back into the hospital, teary eyed, I have little satisfaction, knowing that the bad guy is also dead. Somehow, an eye for an eye just doesn't seem fair. We have lost a vital member of our community, one that unselfishly has given his life for the protection of others.

Terry finally makes it home to find a car parked out in front of her house. It is her dear friend, a sergeant from the police department, and his wife. They spend the night with Terry. Her first night alone.

Later, I would learn that the state of California dedicated the new bridge to our fallen deputy, and one of the volunteers from the Butte County Sheriff Office, Don Hall, took it upon himself to have the cairns placed at both ends of the bridge, a daily reminder of a great person dedicated to the protection of the citizens of Butte County. His name will forever be remembered by all that pass over the bridge entering or leaving Oroville.

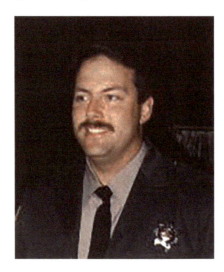

2

FIRST CALL

THIRTY YEARS! OH *my god, has it really been that long?* I wonder as I read a personalized invitation to not only a reunion of the FlightCare staff but also the unveiling of the new FlightCare helicopter. I instantly pick up my phone and text one of my best friends, Marty, the program director of Emergency Services at Enloe. I tell him that I will be there and then ask if he will be giving me a ride in the shiny, new helicopter.

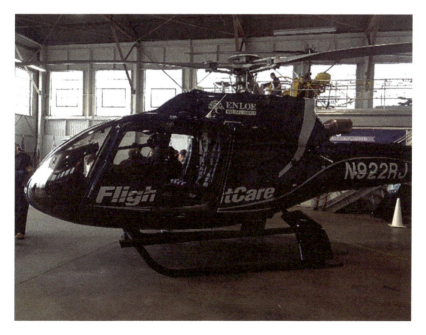

At the reunion, it is so great to meet up with the people that were so important to me and one another in now what seems like a lifetime ago. After the dedication, I continue to bump into friends not seen in over a decade. We all have the same questions, "What are you doing now?" I tell them about working at the fire department and how I have written a book and now starting a second. They all want to know about the stories and even bring up stories long forgotten by myself that I am making mental notes about when Marty approaches me and asks if I'm coming to the EMS symposium next month. I tell him yes, I'll be there, and he promises me a ride if he can work it in.

The November symposium is almost here, and I text Marty one last time to ask if his promise of a ride still stands. He only replies, "Bring your helmet."

Way cool. We all meet up at the symposium, and I mention to Marty that Bruce, one of my EMT battalion chiefs, has also come along with me and it will be great if he can come along with us. "No problem. Just sit tight, enjoy the lectures, and I'll let you know when we can go."

Bruce and I have been listening to the lectures and hearing the helicopter coming and going all day. It has been very busy for them, and I'm starting to think the ride may not happen when there is a text from Marty. "Get over to the ED now!"

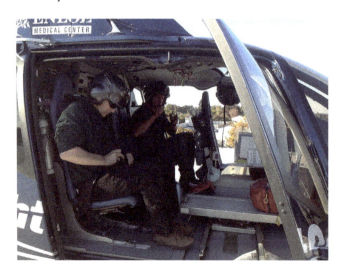

Bruce and I don't have to be told twice; we grab our gear and race over to the ED and are met up with Marty, who tells us that he has to be somewhere else but Roger will be going for fuel and is expecting us. We ride up the elevator to the roof and meet up with Roger, who had just started working here my last year before I left, and we check out the new helicopter and get buckled in.

The new helicopter is incredible! It's an Airbus EC-130 EcoStar. And Enloe has the designation to be the first to use the new EC-130 for emergency medical service. I quickly notice how much more room there is from the A-Star, more visibility, quieter, all-glass display.

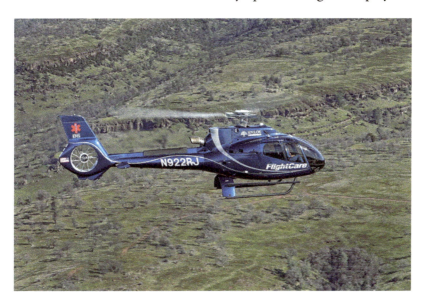

Roger takes us out to the airport and points out some more of the features, then takes on a demonstration flight that takes us around Butte County, and before we know it, we are returning to the airport for more fuel.

After returning to our seats in the symposium, Bruce and I find ourselves not paying much attention when he asks, "Do you remember your first call?" I think for about a second before answering him, "Yes, I do. I can never forget it." Then in a whispering voice, I start telling him the story that started my career in EMS.

FIRST CALL

I made it! After being a driver on the fire department ambulance and helping the EMTs on scenes over the last several years as a first responder, I have finally finished the EMT class and have the new Northern California Emergency Medical Services (Nor Cal EMS) EMT-1 card in my hand.

The state has just recently gotten involved in tracking EMTs, and to give you a little idea how new all this is, I am Nor Cal EMS, EMT number 00157. The current EMT numbers are up into the tens of thousands.

I am really excited about my new certification. Responding with the fire department over the last few years, I have already gained a lot of knowledge. Now I just can't wait for my first call to be the primary caregiver in the back of the ambulance.

Confucius or one of those philosophers once said, "Be careful for what you wish for!"

The fire department is equipped with an ambulance that, for its day, is state-of-the-art. It is a type II Chevrolet Suburban. It has a raised roof and is four-wheel drive, which is fairly rare in the seventies and eighties. I have been driving it for several years and know it really is an ideal rig for our area. We are in the high Sierras, about an hour north of Lake Tahoe. We commonly respond into the national forest for vehicle accidents, logging accidents, and injuries associated with all the summer camping, fishing, and hunting weekend activities. Then in the winter, with an average snowfall of around three to ten feet, vehicle and snowmobile accidents are a common occurrence.

There is no hospital in Sierraville, where we are stationed; the closest is in Loyalton, thirteen miles to the east. But this is pretty much a quick stop. The doctor will come from his house, evaluate the patient, maybe put an IV into them, then tell us to load them back up and either head to Truckee or Reno. By the time I attended paramedic school, I already had more trauma experience than all the rest of my class put together.

The one big drawback this suburban has is its gas tank. It can make a round trip to Reno and back only if you are headed that way at the beginning of the call. If you have to drive out into the forest to pick up a patient and then head to Reno, you need gas to get home.

ON THE GO

My father, the fire chief of the department, and I both have stashes of cash, usually a twenty-dollar bill, tucked away for one of those 2:00 a.m. calls and needing to take on some gas to get home. There is nothing worse than getting to Reno, dropping off the patient, driving to a gas station, and finding someone has used the cash and has not replaced it yet. I don't know exactly how many times we've had to beg for gas money to get home, but I can tell you it has been more than once.

The day finally comes. I am scheduled to be the EMT on the rig for the entire twenty-four hours. I spend the entire morning at the firehouse and meticulously go through all the boxes and first-out bags. I want to make sure I know that everything is in its place but also want to refresh my recall of where different items are. I will set a bag down on the gurney, study it from the outside, quiz myself as to what should be in each compartment, then open it up to see if I am correct.

I hang around the fire department most of the day, and by evening, I start to think my day in the limelight will never come. By five o'clock, I finally give up for the evening and go home. As I sit back in my recliner, dozing off, running different scenarios through my head, I am jolted from my semiconsciousness by the pager suddenly going off. I don't even think I've pulled the handle back to put the chair back into its upright position. All I know is, I am out of the chair and almost to my truck before the beeping stops. As I race down to the fire station, the dispatcher starts relaying information to us. We are being requested to Sierra City to pick up a medical patient complaining of chest pain.

Sierra City isn't in our primary response area, but we soon learned that the ambulance in Downieville is already out on a call and we are the next closest.

As I arrive at the fire station, the fire chief is already there and is opening the doors. I have worked with him for many years and also know he is one of the first EMTs in the first class held north of Sacramento. It will be good knowing he is in the rig with me, in case I have questions or have a problem.

FIRST CALL

We both buckle into the seats, and he pulls the rig out of the engine bay. As we start our trip over to Sierra City, we discuss how long it may take us to get there and, even more important, how long it may take us to get to a hospital. The Downieville ambulance that usually covers this area will usually transport the patient down the canyon to Grass Valley. Neither one of us really wants to go there as we don't even know where the Grass Valley hospital is, and we are pretty sure that the entire ride will be well over two hours. We finally come up with a plan to encourage the patient to be transported back to Loyalton. This in itself will be a transport from the scene to the hospital of around an hour and a half.

We quickly cross the flatlands of Sierra Valley and start up the hill to Yuba Pass. To get to Sierra City, we leave the valley floor at 5,000 feet, climb to 7,100 feet at the summit, then descend to 4,000 feet in Sierra City. All this is done in approximately 35 miles. As you can guess, it is incredibly steep and very windy. There are many turns marked at 15 to 20 miles per hour. A lot of the traffic accidents we go to are from people going too fast on this stretch of road and either driving off one of the turns or a logging truck losing its brakes and rolling over on a turn.

As we climb to the summit, I can tell the chief is driving the suburban like it is a sports car. He doesn't drive much, as he is usually in the back. His foot is to the floor every time he comes out of a turn, and you can hear the large four-barrel guzzling gas, then slamming on the brakes as he enters the next turn. By the time we crest the summit, I can tell the engine is starting to heat up from all the aggressive driving, and the gas gauge, one of the biggest gauges on the dash, is already below three-fourths of a tank, close to one-half, and I am starting to wonder if we will even have enough gas to make it back to Loyalton.

Starting down the west side of the mountain is proving to be much better on gas mileage, but that gain is being transferred to the brakes. We are flying down the hill, and he is slamming the brakes on at each turn. I feel I should speak up and politely ask if he could *SLOW DOWN* but decide that since he is the chief and I'm just a newbie EMT, what do I know?

ON THE GO

Just as we are entering the outskirts of Sierra City, I can definitely smell the distinct order of hot brakes. I have been on the radio and in contact with one of the Sierra City firefighters. He is telling us that they are just off the main highway at a motel. He is also saying that he will be standing at the entrance and will flag us down when we approach, as neither one of us is very familiar with this town.

The speed limit through town is 25 miles per hour, but it is obvious that the chief doesn't really care, as we are somewhere around 55 to 60. Soon, I spot the reflections from a fire department jacket standing on the side of the road and can make out arms waving in the air at us. As I point to the rapidly approaching flagger, I tell the chief, "I think this is it." My finger is still pointing at the firefighter and tracks the man from the front of the ambulance all the way to the rear as we fly past him. By the time my finger has passed by the chief and is now pointing toward the direction we just came from, I look back at my driver and can see a change in his face. I take a few seconds, noticing that we really aren't slowing, and ask, "Did you see him?" It takes him a moment, but he finally replies to me, keeping his eyes forward. "Having a little trouble stopping this thing!"

Crap! I think to myself, as I now know what I had been worried about throughout this roller-coaster ride over the hill. The brakes are beyond hot, and there is no way he is going to be able to stop this thing. I lean forward, looking out the mirror outside of my door, and as we pass through the city, I can make out a definite trail of blue smoke following us through the quiet mountain town.

At this point, I really have no idea what the chief has in mind for us. I decide to just sit back and watch dear ole dad sweat. He has pulled the transmission out of drive and has been downshifting it to get the engine to assist us in slowing down. By the time he gets it slow enough to shift it into first gear, we are now down to around 25 miles per hour. I am not too familiar with the town but do know there is a turn up ahead that, if he can make to, will put us on a road that immediately goes uphill. Due to the simple rules of gravity, this should bring us to a stop. If he misses this road, I believe we will be on a freewheel to the next town of Downieville, about twenty miles farther down the road.

The chief goes for it and, with the tires squealing, almost slides the suburban ninety degrees to the right onto the dirt road. Almost immediately, the rig comes to a stop as the front starts up the grade. Now with the vehicle at a dead stop, blue smoke coming from all four wheels, I turn to him and ask, "So now what?" He turns to look at me and, for a few moments, says nothing. As we sit there, we discuss our options. "Well, it is uphill back to the motel where the patient is. We could creep along, and by the time we assess the patient and load him up, the brakes should be cool enough for the trip to Loyalton." Just saying it brings back into my thought process that we still have to go back over the mountain pass and down the other side back to the valley, and this is the steeper and longer portion of the mountain. But I think he has learned his lesson and will be taking it much slower down the hill.

We decide to go for it, and the chief backs the rig onto the highway and we start back up the road to where we had flown by the firefighter, leaving nothing but a blue cloud of smoking asbestos. As we now slowly approach the man, we can see he is right where we left him, only now he isn't waving his arms to flag us down, but as we come to a stop, he only lifts his arms out to his side as if to say, "What the hell?"

As we slow then stop, I open the window and ask, "Excuse me, sir, did you call for an ambulance?" I can see there is no humor in his facial expression. He is already mad about having to wait longer for us to get there instead of the local ambulance, and then the smoking fly-by doesn't help matters. I then try to focus onto something else and ask him where the patient is. He points down a very steep driveway and tells us, "He's in number 11." Looking down the driveway, I can make out a couple of rescue vehicles and several cars that I'm guessing belong to other tenants of the motel. Knowing the brakes are still way too hot to attempt driving down into the parking lot, knowing that it will be fairly probable that we will only stop by running either into a parked fire or personnel car or into one of the rooms, we decide to just grab our gear and walk down the driveway to the room.

I ask the firefighter to help me, and after pulling a few things out of the back of the ambulance, we make our way down the driveway and into the patient's room. As I enter, I can see a couple other personnel dressed in fire turnout gear, and in front of them is a man in his early sixties. I walk up to the fire personnel and patient, now back into my mind-set of being a medical provider, knowing there are no EMTs in this town. The closest ones are on the ambulance in Downieville. I introduce myself for everyone to hear. "Hi, I'm an EMT!" I'm hoping everyone will be very impressed, but to my surprise, they just start in with giving me a report on the patient. I could have told them I was the tooth fairy, and I think I would have gotten the same response. It is around midnight, and all these people have one thing on their mind, getting home and back to bed.

I take the report from the fire personnel, then introduce myself to the patient and start in with the usual questions. As this is my very first patient, I am going through my memorized list of questions as if I'm taking my final exam in class and don't want to miss a single question: "What's your name?" "How old are you?" "When did this pain start?" "Can you describe it to me?" "Have you taken anything for it?" "Does it radiate?" "On a scale of one to ten…" I suddenly notice the patient isn't talking. "Is there something wrong?" I ask. The patient then replies back, "Are you just going to keep asking questions, or are you going to wait for any answers?" He is absolutely right; I have fallen into a classroom-taught memorization of all the questions you need to ask to get through my final checkoff during skills testing. You must recite all the proper questions, but in class, they really don't teach you that you must wait for an answer to each question before you go onto the next. In the future, I will see this same trap in many EMT, paramedics, and nursing students.

I know my patient is right and excuse myself and start over, this time writing down his answers to all the questions I have been asking. The Sierra City firefighters already have the patient on oxygen and have been taking his vital signs and are taking one last set just as my chief walks into the door. I stand up and ask him how we are going to get the patient out to the ambulance. He tells me that the brakes have cooled enough that he's been able to bring the rig down into the parking lot and just want to know if we can walk him out or if we should bring in the gurney. Being that this is a chest pain patient and he may be having a heart attack, I ask him to bring the gurney in.

Before long, with some assistance from a couple of Sierra City firefighters, they roll the gurney into the room, and in no time, we have him loaded up and are securing him back into the rig. As we are doing this and I am climbing in, I can still smell the hot brakes, but at least the smoke has discontinued.

As the chief is closing the doors to the back of the rig, leaving me inside the rear with the patient, I can hear some of the firefighters giving the chief a bad time about his driving skills. I smile a bit, then unsmile, as I think of the ride off the other side of Yuba Pass. I decide to focus my attention back to the patient. I switch over the oxygen to the vehicle O_2, take a set of vital signs, then enter into a discussion with him on where he is from and what he is doing in the area. He starts in by telling me he is from the Sacramento area and he comes up each year to enjoy the mountains and do some fishing.

As we leave Sierra City and head up the mountain, I can already tell the ride is much more pleasurable. The chief is taking his time, and as we start our descent into the valley side of the mountain, I feel the rig slow, as he has pulled the transmission out of drive into second gear to engine-brake his way down the hill.

The driver's compartment and patient compartment in the suburban are separated by a sliding window that can be accessed by either side. I notice the chief has pulled the windows closed and has probably turned on the radio to listen to some music on the long drive to the hospital in Loyalton. As we continue our descent down the hill, I watch as the windy road is slowly putting our patient to sleep, and I continue to monitor his vital signs and have turned down the lights.

In the seventies and eighties, ambulances have an option of having a blue light in the rear. I really like this light, as we do a lot of long-distance, late-night transports, and it is very comforting for the patient not to have the bright white overhead lights shining into their eyes. The drawback is, if someone is losing consciousness or has gone into cardiac arrest and coded, you can't tell if they are cyanotic—they will always look blue. So to combat this, you will either check their pulse occasionally or wake them to see how they are doing. This is exactly what I am doing, feeling for a pulse when I check vital signs and occasionally asking, "How are you doing?"

Nearing the bottom of the hill, I decide to check his vital signs one last time before we start across the valley, which means picking up speed on the straighter roads, which causes more noise, vibration, and rough ride at the higher speeds and makes it harder to hear in the stethoscope. I reach down and feel for a radial pulse at the patient's wrist and, after repositioning my grasp several times, become puzzled, as I can't find the pulse that I have been using for the last forty-five minutes. It simply seems to have disappeared. Puzzled, I slowly move my hand up to the patient's neck and feel for his carotid pulse. After a couple of attempts, I start to become worried as I can't find anything. I am now starting to wonder if it is just me, the newbie EMT, or if something is truly wrong. I then decide to wake the patient and start gently nudging him and, with, at first, a soft voice, ask, "Hey, hey, are you okay?" As I do not get any answer, my soft and gentle voice becomes much louder, with a slight quiver of panic, as I am now shaking him and hollering, "HEY, WAKE UP!"

Pure panic now sets in. My patient isn't responding. I turn to the front of the compartment and, with a monstrous banging of my fist on the sliding window, scream, "HE'S CODED!" The fire chief, who has slipped into a pleasant humming along with the music, running mindless thoughts through his head, almost comes out of his seat with my screaming and thunderous banging of the window. In a scared-out-of-his-mind almost-panic, his flight-or-fight responses cause him to not only try to jump away from the loud, screaming demon right behind his head, but in doing so, he also makes a jerk of the steering wheel, which sends me flying off my little jump seat in the back of the ambulance as it responds to the violent steering input. Then, as the chief struggles to bring the rig back under control, hits the brakes, and regains control of his bowels, I am tossed around in the back like a tennis ball in a clothes dryer. After some impressive driving and keeping the rig on the road, he is finally able to slide the window open just as I am picking myself off the floor. He asks, "What?"

Yelling back at him now through the open window, I rub the side of my head that hit something during the event. "I think he coded."

To my surprise, I hear a voice coming from the rear of the vehicle asking, "Hey, what is going on?"

"Are you still alive?" I ask, totally stunned to see the patient now looking at me and answering questions.

"What do you mean am I still alive? Of course I'm still alive."

I move back to the bench next to the patient and feel his wrist to find that I once again have the thumping of the pulse that I have been monitoring. And now I don't understand what has happened.

"Everything okay back there?" the chief asks through the open window.

"Yes, we're okay, keep going," I reply.

The chief, shaking his head, reaches up and slides the window closed once again. I start up a conversation with my patient and decide that I am not going to let him sleep any more on our trip. I turn off the blue lights and switch on the white lights, which, I can tell, the patient doesn't like, but at this point, I don't care.

The rest of the trip to the Loyalton hospital is uneventful, and as we wheel the patient into the ER, I report off to the nurse and sheepishly tell her that at one point, I couldn't wake him or feel a pulse. In reality, I am blaming myself that I panicked and I'm sure that the patient was probably fine and that the whole event was probably my fault. Then I tell myself that I think I've failed with my first patient as an EMT.

After we load the gurney back into the ambulance and restock the used equipment, the two of us start our trip back to the fire department in Sierraville. As we cruise along in the early hours of the morning, I can tell the chief wants to say something about my panic episode, and finally looking at him, I say, "Go ahead. I know you want to give me shit about pounding on the window, scaring the crap out of you." Laughing, he then tells me that was in fact not the first time that had happened, then I bring up the hot brake issue and that it was only by the grace of God that we somehow survived the ride to Sierra City. By the time we're back into the bay at the fire station, we are both laughing, and as the chief is turning out the lights and I'm closing the door, we come to an agreement that maybe we should keep the events of this evening to ourselves.

Surprisingly, a few days later, we transport another patient to the Loyalton hospital, and the doctor takes me aside to tell me about the patient we had brought in from Sierra City a few nights past. He goes on to tell me that they have admitted him for observation and have placed him on a cardiac monitor. They were surprised when he went into ventricular tachycardia a couple of times, each time losing his pulse and becoming unconscious. Later that morning, they send him off to the larger hospital in Reno for a cardiologist.

It was reassuring to know that indeed, when I couldn't find his pulse, and not having the luxury of a cardiac monitor, I hadn't failed, that the patient's heart indeed had stopped pumping and that was why I couldn't feel his pulse. It was a valuable lesson in my early days of what would be over a forty-year career.

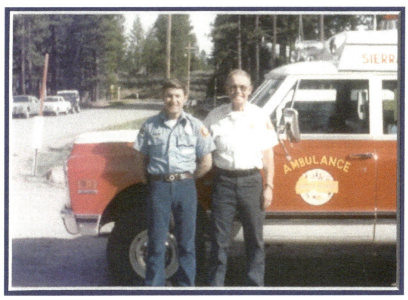

The author with his father, the Chief, and the Suburban ambulance.

3

HIGHWAY 50

IN MY EARLY days of being on the helicopter in Chico, I live in Fair Oaks, one of the many cities that surround Sacramento. Although my normal shift is from 6:00 p.m. to 6:00 a.m., this is my final of six nights working, and it has been incredibly foggy for the last two nights, and I will be off for eight days starting this morning. Even the day shift hasn't been able to fly anywhere, as the fog has been so thick and hasn't let up during the day.

Around midnight, after several hours of some serious whining, I am finally able to talk the charge nurse into letting me go home early. There is no way the helicopter is going out, and the ED has been so slow that many of the staff have gone to their secret spots to sleep for a few hours. As I walk across the street to the parking lot to look for my truck, I can't believe how foggy it really is. After finding my truck, I throw in my bags and start out driving through the dense fog. I have planned to leave Chico when I get off this morning, so all my stuff from the apartment is already in the truck, and it is ready for the drive home.

A couple of hours later, as I am entering the outskirts of Sacramento, I am surprised to see the fog isn't as bad down here. By the time I turn off of I-5 onto Highway 50 to head east to Fair Oaks, it is clear, and I can see stars. This also lets me finally relax in my seat after the two hours of intense night-fog driving, waiting for that unknown obstacle or gremlin to pop up right in front of you at any moment. Within twenty minutes, I have turned the radio up and find myself almost becoming too relaxed, risking falling asleep.

To fight this, I crack the window open a little to let some of the cool night air into the truck, and knowing I only have another ten to fifteen minutes before I'm home, I press on.

As I'm leaving Sacramento, I find myself in the middle of five lanes of the freeway almost all by myself. It is almost a little eerie. I can make out some taillights about a mile in front of me and nothing behind me. My mind is nowhere to be found. It has drifted off into someplace distant, thinking of some of the things I would like to get done on my days off when another part of my mind is telling me to wake up! I bring myself back together and find myself trying to understand what it is that my eyes are focusing on and my mind can't compute.

At first, all I see are taillights, but they are spinning around, changing with white headlights then back to red taillights, when suddenly they change from being horizontal to vertical, one over the top of the other. I instinctively tap the clutch pedal that shuts off the cruise control, and I can feel the truck decelerating. At the same time, I'm leaning forward, trying to make sense of what I'm seeing. As the truck is slowing but now close enough for my headlights to light up the area, I am suddenly faced with a full-size van sitting on its side in the middle of the freeway. The wheels on the upper side are still spinning, and there is some smoke coming from the front of it.

Although I don't totally understand why this van has decided to flip over onto its side in the middle of an empty freeway, I come to a stop, leaving my headlights aimed at the van to light it up. After turning on my emergency flashers, I grab my fire extinguisher and run up to the van, knowing that there is probably someone inside, and I want to make sure it isn't going to catch fire. As I walk around to the front, I don't see any flames, but there is some smoke coming from under the hood, so I aim my extinguisher through the grill and into the engine compartment the best that I can and squeeze the trigger. The dry chemical blows out and into the front of the van, covering everything in a yellow dust. I then move it around into a few different places to try to cover more area. When I have almost exhausted its full content, I step back and take a good look at the van. I am surprised to see that the entire front of the van is destroyed, smashed in, as if it hit something. At that point, I pull my flashlight out of my pocket, and slowly turning, shining the light in a sweep across the freeway, I stop when it lights up a second car about fifty feet down the road. I turn back to the van, and walking up to the windshield and shining the light inside, all I see are empty front seats. Banging on the windshield with the butt end of the light, I yell, "Hello, is there anyone in here?"

Almost immediately, a voice answers, "Yes, I'm in here. I need help!" I then ask if he is by himself, and he answers yes. Standing back, looking at the van on its side, I know if the rear doors don't open, it will be a problem getting to the driver. I ask if he thinks he is injured, and he tells me that he knows his arm is broken but otherwise he thinks he is okay. Thinking quickly and knowing I still need to go check out the car, I tell him that the best thing he can do right now is to just stay where he is. The van is a safe place, and fire personnel will help him get out when they get here.

As he agrees, I turn and jog down to the car, shining my light at it as I approach, looking for any hazards, like fuel spilling. I can see the car is still upright, but the entire front of it is destroyed. The one thing that really catches my eye is that the front bumper is pushed all the way up to the windshield and there is nothing in front of that. The entire motor and front axle have been pushed back and down, part of it under the car, part of it inside the car. I make a quick circle around the car, starting on the passenger side, shining my light into it, looking for patients. I really can't tell if there is anyone in the front passenger seat, as it is now just twisted metal. Looking in the rear, I see the rear seats are empty. As I arrive back at the location where the driver's door used to be, I shine my light in and can see a body slumped over what was the steering wheel. The dash is pushing the man's torso tightly against the back of the seat. There is a large wound on his forehead, and a flap of skin is hanging down over one of his eyes. Blood is everywhere. I also notice that his left arm is bent around 180 degrees at the mid humerus area, as if he has two elbows. I have seen many dead people in many car accidents, and from my survey of the car and now what I'm looking at, what used to be a driver, I think in my mind, *This guy is dead!*

I also know not to take anything for granted. I don a pair of gloves that I always keep as spares in my flight suit as I look for a route to reach in and try to locate a pulse. The front and driver's side of the car are so mangled that I have to slowly pick the route that I will put my arm into this twisted mess and try to reach the driver. I can tell that he is not breathing but still don't know if he has a pulse. I start working my right arm through the broken glass, pieces of dash, jagged metal, and finally, my shoulder fully pressed up against the outside of the wreck. At my full reach, I can feel the bloody side of his face. I slowly slide my hand down to the area in his neck where the carotid artery should be, telling myself, *If he doesn't have a pulse, I'm done and can go back to the guy in the van.*

I try and try but simply can't get my fingers to the side of his neck. *Time for plan B.* I decide to attempt to open his airway and see if he is breathing. If not, I can say I've tried everything I can do and go back to help the guy in the van. The driver's head is bent over to the front, his chin resting over the steering wheel and is almost wrapped all the way over the steering wheel, touching his chest. The only thing I can do with one hand is to grab his hair and pull up. I work my hand to the top of his head, and making sure I have as much hair as I can grab, I pull his head up and back, lifting his chin off the steering wheel and into an open-airway position. Almost instantly, I can hear the patient taking in a huge gasp of air. At first, I am surprised, then think to myself that this might actually be some trapped air escaping or some type of last, dying, agonal breath. I continue to hold his head in an inline position, and after about ten seconds, he takes another gasp of air.

"Shit!" Now I'm frozen. I know I am going to have to stay here in this position to do one of three things. One, wait for him to quit breathing altogether. Two, wait for him to possibly wake up. Or three, wait for the local emergency responder to show up so I can turn this entire mess over to them and continue my trip home. Either way, I'm now stuck here. I know, in my current position, with my arm fully extended, holding his head, I will die from fatigue in a matter of minutes. I attempt to wiggle my upper torso around, and finally, I'm able to find a way to rest my arm a little and have been able to slide some loose car parts under a part of my arm to help support it. Now I just need to wait for the cavalry.

Within the first few minutes, a couple of other cars have pulled up, and some Good Samaritans are asking me what they can do. "Run to my pickup, and in the back is an orange trauma bag. Go grab it!" I yell out to him. I tell one of the other people to go talk to the van driver, instructing them, "Just leave him in the van but talk to him. Let him know he is safe and help is on its way."

Before long, the man has returned with my trauma bag, and I ask him to open it, telling him where to look. He is able to finally find me an oral airway. As he gives it to me and I hold it in my left hand, I wonder, *How in the world am I going to get this thing in*? Then it strikes me. I have nothing better to do. It takes a few minutes, and with the help of the Samaritan holding the flashlight, somehow, I not only have been able to work the airway up to the patient's face but have also actually been able to place it into his mouth. As soon as I have done this, I can tell it is easier to maintain his head in a position to allow air to now flow in and out. The patient still isn't regaining consciousness, but I can tell he is pinker than when I first walked up and found him in a deathly color of blue.

It seems likes hours, but in reality, I'm sure it has only been around five to ten minutes before the first fire engine pulls up alongside of the car. I watch as the captain steps out of the engine and works his way over to me, shining his flashlight first on the wreckage. Then as he turns to talk to me, he shines his light first at my face then down to my feet and back up to my face once again. It suddenly strikes me that I'm still in my flight suit. He then asks, "Are you a LifeFlight nurse?" LifeFlight is the flight program based at the University of California Davis Medical Center here in Sacramento, and actually, it is only about five miles from where we are. I can see how he can easily mistake me for one of their crew as we are in their city and we wear the same royal blue flight suits. "No, I'm a flight paramedic from Chico," I tell him. At that point, he shines his flashlight at my name tag and can read my name and FLIGHT PARAMEDIC, ENLOE FLIGHTCARE. Looking back up at me, he then asks, "What do you need?" I tell him about the patient in the van and then ask him to find someone to relieve me as my arm is killing me. Pausing for a second, he then tells me that since I'm a paramedic and they are only EMTs and he needs all his crew to start with extrication, I'll have to wait for the ambulance crew to relieve me.

I understand this and also know that a paramedic in Sacramento is still an intimidating thing as there is no such thing as a paramedic in Sacramento City or county. All the fire departments and ambulances are still running with EMT-Is and EMT-IIs. "Okay" I agree, but then ask, "Can you find out the ETA of the ambulance?" He agrees, then stepping away, I can hear him radioing his dispatch, asking for another engine and an ETA on the ambulance. As he is walking away to talk to his crew, I do yell out for him to have someone bring me some oxygen so I can put it on the patient. He nods and joins up with his crew.

As one of the fire crew helps me apply the oxygen, I can see the second engine pulling up, and with it, an ambulance. *Finally*, I think. *I'll turn this guy over to them and get the hell out of here.* The ambulance comes to a stop, and I watch as a young girl steps out of the passenger side as her partner gets out of the driver's side and makes a run down the freeway for the van. As she walks up to me, just as the fire captain did, I can see a slightly confused look on her face, then she shines her light on my name tag. I decide to introduce myself and give her a report. I do this, and just as I'm finishing and hoping she will take over for me, she speaks up, telling me, "Well, because you're a paramedic and I am just an EMT-II, and this is a critical patient, I don't feel comfortable taking over his care from you."

"Really," I say, then add, "I really haven't done anything that isn't in your scope of practice."

She then tells me that it is their policy that in situations like this, I will have to stay with the patient and ride with her to the hospital. *Bullshit!* I think to myself. *There is no policy like that.* I know better. She can take over, but she just doesn't want to. I also know I do not want to spend the rest of my night riding in an ambulance to the medical center then trying to find a ride back to my truck, abandoning it in the middle of Highway 50. But I also know that I'm not going to argue with her, so now knowing she has dumped this call onto me, telling me this is my patient, I tell her, "Call LifeFlight."

Staring at me, she finally asks, "What do you mean? We can do the transport."

I then tell her, "I'm in charge, right?" She nods. "This is my patient, right?" She nods again. "Good, then I'm telling you to call the helicopter and we'll fly this guy to the medical center."

Now she knows that her attempt to pull one over on me will cost the ambulance company the revenue from the lost transport. She radios the request in, and as she finishes, I ask her to prepare an IV. At that point, she stays with me, and working together with the fire department, we are finally able to gain more access to the patient after the roof of the car is cut off. As they are pulling the dash off the patient, he is now starting to moan and move around a little. I try to talk to him, telling him that he has been in an accident and we are helping him. As I am doing this, my one-sided conversation is interrupted with the sound of a helicopter making an approach onto the freeway.

Within a few more minutes, I can make out the blue suits of the two flight nurses walking up to me, and I recognize one of them. Before I can say anything, she has recognized me, knowing I'm a paramedic from the Chico flight program. She speaks up. "What the hell are you doing here?"

I grin and laugh a little, replying, "Wrong place, wrong time."

She then asks if I was involved in the accident, and I tell her no. I then tell here that the funny thing was, I got off work early because we were fogged in and it was slow and I was just trying to get home. They both laugh, then start asking me about the patient and what happened. I fill them in, and finally having someone to relieve me, I step back and try to shake the cramps out of my arm, wondering how I'm going to shift my truck, because it feels like I have had a stroke and can't move my right arm.

It only takes the fire department another fifteen minutes to finally cut enough of the car away to finally remove the patient. I help secure him to the backboard and assist the crew in carrying him over to the helicopter, and after we slide him in, I say my goodbyes to the crew and start walking back to the wrecked car. I gather up my trauma bag, and as I start walking back to my truck, I stop to talk to one of the CHP officers, who asks me if I saw what happened. I tell him that the first thing I saw was the van flipping over onto its side and I wasn't even aware that there was a second vehicle until I walked up here. At that point, I ask him if he has figured out what happened, and he starts to tell me what he finally came up with after looking at all the skid marks and talking to the van driver.

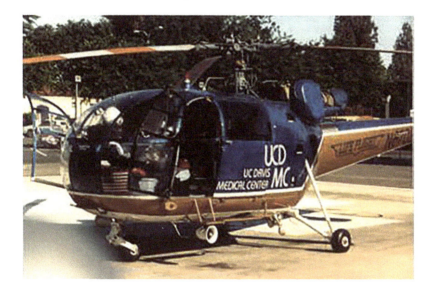

He believes the driver of the car, the very drunk driver, was on his way home from the bar and missed his exit on the freeway. Being of impaired mind and thinking he was the only car out here, he decided it would be easier to just flip a U-turn in the freeway and return to the off-ramp he missed. At that point, the driver of the van told the CHP officer that he really didn't see him coming until just before they collided. Investigating the car, the officer believes that the drunk driver was also driving without his headlights, on and that was why neither the van driver nor I ever saw him. As I listen, I am shaking my head, thinking that if the van hadn't been in front of me, I would have been the next car to come along and might have been the one the car hit head-on. "Unbelievable," I answer, then ask the CHP officer if he needs anything else, and he only asks me for my number in case he needs to get ahold of me. I pull one of my FlightCare business cards out of my pocket and hand it to him. Looking at my card, he then asks, "If you work in Chico, what are you doing here?" I tell him that I actually live here, and turning, I point up the road, saying that I only live about ten minutes up the road in Fair Oaks and I'd really like to get home. He shakes my hand, and as I am putting the trauma bag back into the rear of my truck and shutting the shell door, I look up and watch as the blue-and-gold Alouette helicopter is lifting and flies over me, heading back to the medical center.

I finally make it home and simply throw myself down onto the sofa. All the fatigue of driving in the fog and then the stress of the accident has totally worn me out, and within seconds, I'm out cold.

A week later, I walk back into the ED in Chico on my first day back. As I'm getting a report from the day crew, I feel a tug on my sleeve and turn to find Drena. "What's up?" I ask. Pulling me out into the hallway, she pulls out a newspaper, and opening it, I see the front page of the *Sacramento Bee*. On the cover is a picture of a horrendous accident and a title that reads, "Highway 50 Closed for hours due to head-on accident." Before I can say anything, she raises her finger, pointing to the figure of someone wearing a blue one-piece flight suit bending over into the wrecked car, and she asks, "That is you, isn't it?"

Not sure how to answer that, I study the picture for a moment, then say, "It says UC–Davis LifeFlight was there. Why do you think that is me? You can't see a face."

Now smiling, she looks at me and, more specifically, points to the rear end of the guy in the picture in the blue suit, saying, "I'd know that butt anywhere. It is you! What were you doing there?"

Now laughing, I wrap my arm around her and we slowly walk to the elevator. As we walk, I ask her if she remembers me going home early last week, then tell her about driving up on the accident that happened right in front of me. Knowing this is not the first time something like this has happened to me, she finally says, "You don't get enough trauma here, so you have to go looking for it. What am I going to do with you?"

I smile, saying, "Guess you'll just have to keep a good eye on me and my butt."

We laugh, and as the other crew join us, we say our goodbyes for now and make a possible date to join up for dinner in the cafeteria, just as the elevator doors close.

4

FEATHER RIVER PLANE CRASH

MOST OF THE time, the flights we respond to are to another facility or to rendezvous with an ambulance at the scene of an accident; meaning, there is someone already there. Of the close to 50 percent of the calls we respond to being scene calls, there are those maybe less than 1 percent of our calls that not only are scene calls, putting us right at the accident site, but also even more dramatic and more fun, when we are not only the first responder but also maybe the only responder.

Most of us really like these calls, as they can really challenge us in multiple aspects of our training. Not only do you need to get to the patient, but then you also need to assess them, treat them, extricate them, and then transport them. You must remember that although the helicopter does carry a lot of advanced life support equipment and special equipment such as ventilators and infusion pumps, it carries no extrication equipment. We always rely on the local fire departments for getting their heavy tools such as the Jaws of Life out to rip, cut, and tear cars away from our patients. Not only is there not enough room in the helicopter for this type of equipment, but it also weighs a ton, and in reality, there is only less than 1 percent of our calls that we would maybe need such equipment. So we must rely on what we have with us or call someone to help.

Such is the case this one very hot summer day. Bruce and I meet up in the parking lot, and as we are strolling across the street to the ED, talking about our day and what might happen this evening, we suddenly hear Dennis yelling at us from across the street at the pilot's quarters.

Dennis is fairly new to FlightCare but not new to helicopters. He has been flying for decades, originally earning his wings in the Army, then flying offshore in the Gulf of Mexico. He also has his fixed-wing license and, sometimes on his days off, flies charter planes for a service out of the Chico Airport. He has been a longtime friend of Marty and is fitting in with us really well.

Dennis catches up and joins in with our conversation as we enter the ED and start making our way through the staff, patients, and the gurney garage, trying to get to the lounge to put food in the fridge, get equipment out of our lockers, and check in with the day crew. As I make my way through the ED, a quick look at the patient board behind the charge nurse tells most of the story. The board is full. There is also a stack of charts sitting next to him of patients still in the waiting room, waiting for their turn to be brought back and placed into a bed. This is really not a good way to start the evening; it is swamped.

Just as I start to hum my chant to the flight gods, I spot Drena across the room. She is on the phone, and there are several people trying to talk to her at the same time. I can tell she is being polite and trying to answer all their questions, but I can also see that she isn't looking at them but is looking at me, and as she holds the phone to her ear, her eyes track me as I walk through the room. Then before I disappear around the corner, I flash her a wink, and almost immediately, she smiles and winks back at me.

We enter the lounge to find the day crew sitting at the table. Apparently, they have just gotten back from an interfacility transfer that was a direct admit to one of the ICUs. As we discuss the flight, they fill us in on what may be needed to restock the ship, and slide a bag toward us, telling us that they think everything we need should be in there. As I open the bag to take a quick look, the door opens and the charge nurse sticks his head in, telling us to hurry upstairs, get our checks done, and get back down so we can help out, and without waiting for any answers, he turns and closes the door. I take a quick glance at my watch and see that it is still ten minutes to six, then think I should inform him that we officially aren't even here yet. But the door closes and it is clear he is not interested. I throw up my arms, turning back to the rest of the crew.

"Has it been like this all day?" I ask.

The day crew then answers back, "No. It was fine before we left, but when we got back about thirty minutes ago, we found it like this but knew by the time we got things back together and started our paperwork, you guys would be here and we wouldn't have to deal with it."

I can see a smile on their faces now, knowing that we are more than likely going to have a very busy evening, especially if the pagers never sound.

The three of us finally decide we better stop procrastinating and head up to put the few items back into the helicopter and check out the rest to make sure it is ready to go, in case the flight gods answer our prayers. As we exit the elevator in the ready room on the roof, Bruce and I pull our flight suits off our shoulders and tie the arms around our waist. It must be 110 degrees or hotter out, and we all know the helipad can be much hotter. It is totally exposed to the sun and has been baking in it all day. As we open the door and step out, we can feel the blast of heat, and it makes us pause for a moment. As we continue up the ramp, Dennis adds that we should find a spot to fly to that we can go for a swim. The three of us start coming up with different scenarios and places we could go to that maybe we would have to stage for a while and could jump in the water while we are waiting.

We continue with our check of the ship, and as all of us know, we are pretty much done. We also know that we don't really want to go back down to the ED and be thrown into the pool of patients that are waiting for us. We finally, slowly start our stroll down the ramp, and as we reach the door, Bruce opens it to let us in, and in that very instant, our pagers start beeping.

The three of us pause and stand there, knowing that it more than likely is the evening pager test, but you never know. I believe all three of us have our fingers crossed and are refusing to speak or step into the ready room until we know for sure. The beeping has stopped, and it seems to be taking forever for the words of "Evening pager test" to be announced. The pager finally keys back up, and the announcement comes out. "FlightCare, scene flight. Plane crash above Lime Saddle Marina, heading zero nine zero, thirteen miles. More information to follow."

Somehow, all three of us are already in the helicopter, suits pulled up, helmets on, and the blades are already turning before the end of the dispatch. I have my two-inch tape on my thigh, and as the radio comes online, I key up, telling dispatch that I'm ready to copy the information. Dispatch comes back on and starts telling us that there is a plane down on the north side of Lake Oroville in one of the canyons that leads from Paradise. Also, there is another plane that discovered it and called in the report. They are still circling over the scene, and we can contact them by radio for further instructions. They then give us the contact names and numbers of the fire and ambulances that will be responding, but according to the orbiting plane, he doesn't think anyone can get to it except by helicopter. At that point, we discuss the options of having dispatch put out calls to the CHP and sheriff office to start their helicopters our way.

By the time I get all this information back and forth, I look up from my note-taking and see that we are not just airborne but about halfway to where we think we are going. As I look out my door, I decide that at this point there is really no point in closing it. I will just be opening it again to start looking out and down as we approach the scene, and because of the intense heat of the day, the cooler air blowing into the cabin feels really good.

Soon, Dennis calls out that he can see the plane that is over the scene. He makes a slight bank to the left to correct the course, and as he does this, he makes contact with them on the VHF radio to let them know we are only a few minutes out and to also fill them in that other helicopters have been ordered up. The pilot of the plane informs us that he spotted the plane and at first thought it had maybe been there a while, but then noticed some smoke coming from the engine, and when he decided to drop down closer, he spotted someone lying out on the wing. Dennis acknowledges him as we are now passing the last ridge and will start in under the orbiting plane and start down into the canyon toward the lake.

We are all straining forward, and I'm also looking out the door, all of us trying to spot something resembling a plane crash. We still don't know if this is a plane that lost power and control and simply augured in or if it tried to make a forced landing on some flat area, hoping to keep the plane intact. Is everyone dead? Is everyone okay? All these are unknowns.

As I look out toward the south, I can see that we are right on the northern border of Lake Oroville and wonder if the plane might actually be in the water. I don't have to wait any longer. As I look out of the open door and glance down to the north, I can see the river that is flowing down the canyon into the lake, and there on the embankment, with one wing partially submerged, is the plane.

"There it is!" I yell out over the intercom, pointing out the door at the same time.

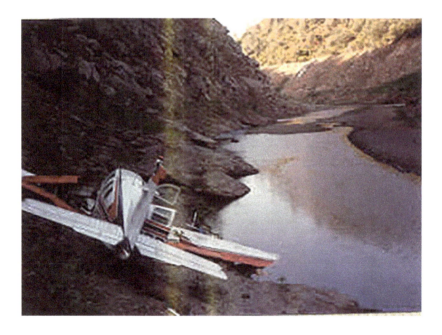

Dennis immediately banks the helicopter over to the left, toward the direction I'm pointing, and within seconds, we are over the scene. We make one quick radio call to dispatch that we are indeed over a plane on the shore of the lake and can see one person out on the wing partially in the water and he doesn't appear to be moving. We also inform them that we will be descending to check for survivors, and we may also lose any contact with them until we get back up to the ridgeline. As we start to settle farther into the canyon, dispatch acknowledges our transmission, then quickly fills us in that the CHP helicopter is en route and about thirty minutes out and the sheriff's helicopter has about a forty-five minute ETA, as they are coming from Sacramento.

As we descend in a circle, we try to not only check for wires that might be crossing the canyon but also try to decide where we should land. The embankment next to the plane is clear of trees or debris but is fairly steep. The other side of the river is all rocks and not an option. We finally agree, if we have any chance to land at all, it may be on a sandbar right in the middle of the river. About one football-field length down the drainage from the plane, the river widens out and looks fairly shallow and has created a sandbar in the middle that is about thirty feet across and about a hundred feet long. The only catch is, How soft is the sand? We really don't know and will only be guessing until we actually try to set down on it.

We make our approach to the northern part of the sand, closest to the wreck, for two reasons. First, we won't have to walk as far, and second, this will leave room for the other helicopters if we need them. Dennis is slowing the ship, and I'm leaning out with one foot on the skid, looking forward and down. The two of us have been talking about the limits of the sand and what he will feel comfortable with. If it is too soft and the ship is either settling to one side or sinking, he will just pull back up and we will do a hover off-load of the two of us. All in agreement, we are now about five feet over the sand, and he has stopped all forward momentum and letting the helicopter settle straight down. I'm now looking straight down and concentrating on the height above the sand, and I'm worried about this being too soft for us to land, which will only complicate us getting any patients out of here.

As we descend, I start calling out our altitude. "Four feet, three feet, two feet, one foot!" Then you can feel the rear of the skids making contact with the sand. Dennis is hesitant about putting the full weight of the helicopter down until he feels it out a little, and as he is slightly bouncing the ship off the sand, I can see that it only appears to be settling in a couple of inches. He then puts the helicopter down, holding a little pressure up on the collective, and I watch for a few seconds, then finally tell him, "I don't see it sinking at all. I think we will be good." Dennis then drops the collective all the way down, putting the entire weight of the helicopter on the sand. I quickly unsnap my harness and jump out, looking under the entire ship without unhooking my helmet so I can keep in verbal contact with him in case I see something. After a few more seconds, I stand up and tell him "We're good!" then I pull off my helmet and start arranging equipment to take with us.

Bruce and I have grabbed our bags and, throwing them over our shoulders like backpacks, decide to not take the gurney at this time as we are still not sure how we are going to get to the plane and don't want to be weighed down with too much equipment. We start out from the sandbar, and what I have noticed from the air is that there seems to be a shallow flow to our left that will take us across the first part of the river. We can then walk up the opposite embankment until we are directly across from the plane, then wade the main river. As we start the first part of our journey through, the water is only about knee-deep, and we forge it for about ten feet. We climb out onto the embankment and start up about one hundred feet and stop as we are now directly across from the plane. We take a moment to try to see how deep the water is and how fast the current is here, and looking across at the plane, I can see the man on the wing and yell at him, "Just hang on! We will be there in a minute!" I can also see a film on the water and know this must either be fuel or oil coming from the plane.

We finally decide to just go for it, and I volunteer to go first. I decide that the worst-case scenario is that I will be washed downstream by the current but should just end up by the helicopter and would have to attempt my journey again. I step into the water, and after a couple of steps, I am up to my waist, then midchest. I am attempting to hold my medical bags over my head to keep them dry, then within a few more steps, I can tell I am climbing up, as it is getting shallower and I can drop the bags back down to my waist. As I approach the plane, I can see the man holding on to the wing and that he is also in the water up to his waist and seems to be clinging on for dear life, and even from my distance, I can see fear in his eyes, which tells me that he is really scared. I turn around to tell Bruce to come across but notice I don't have to; he has watched me wade the river and is now only a few steps behind me.

As I reach the plane, I can see the passenger door open and can hear moaning coming from inside. The man outside is on the opposite side of the wing from me, and as I pause to take all this in, I ask him if he is okay. He quickly responds to me that he cannot move his legs. Now I know why he has the look of terror in his eyes—he is afraid that if he loses his grip from the wing and slips into the water, he will be washed away, and since he cannot move his legs, he can't swim and very well may drown.

I know I should go help him, reassure him that we are here to help, but I also know that I need to triage whoever else may be in the plane. I then ask the man if he can just hang on a few more minutes as we check out the others, and he tells us that he understands. I think just having us here has added a lot of comfort to his anxiety. He knows now that if he starts to drift downstream, we will jump in and pull him out.

I stick my head into the already-open front door of the plane, and I'm totally taken aback by what I see. Not only is there still someone at the pilot's seat, but behind him, the six-seater plane seems to be full. I can tell just by looking that the pilot is unconscious but still alive; he is breathing, slumped over the controls, and there is blood everywhere. It is hard to determine any more about the passengers in the rear. We are going to have to open up the rear doors and take a better look.

As I pull my head out of the front of the plane, I fill Bruce in with what is going on, and I can also see Dennis wading across the river to join us. Between the three of us, we come up with a plan. Bruce will go ahead and start treating the man on the wing. Dennis is very familiar with these planes and can help me with the doors and move seats inside the plane if needed so we can better evaluate the other patients.

With our plan in motion, Dennis and I go to the side of the plane where we find the rear passenger doors, and with a little struggle at first, Dennis is able to get the two doors open. As we start to open them, it suddenly feels as if someone is pushing on them. I brace myself against the door I'm holding and peek around to the inside. There I find a woman in her midforties, unconscious, leaning against the door. Dennis immediately helps me, and between the two of us, we are able to slowly open the doors, then gently remove the woman out onto the ground. I know at this point we are really going to need more people to help. I was only expecting one or two patients, but at this time, I may have five or six, and so far, the only three I have had contact with are all critical.

We have been thrust into a very difficult situation. Bruce and I each have a critical patient, and we still haven't triaged all the others. As much as I would like and feel compelled to help the woman, I know I have to continue triaging the patients remaining in the plane. I finally decide that I have to leave the woman on her own for the time being; if she goes into respiratory or cardiac arrest, I'll just have to let her go. There are others to take care of.

I inform Dennis that we have to get back inside the plane and I'll need his help. The two of us then return to the plane and take a look inside. In the rear seat, I can see a young girl, maybe in her midteens, staring at me with wide worried eyes, and I ask how she is doing. She tells me that she thinks her left arm is broken. I can also see a laceration on her forehead, but it is really good to know she is alert. I tell her we will get back to her in a few minutes, then ask if there is someone sitting next to her. She looks down next to her and tells me that yes, her little brother is sitting there. From my viewpoint, I am not able to see any little brother, as the middle seat still has another patient lying across it. She then tells me that he is in a car seat. *Crap!* I think to myself. I really don't want to deal with an infant but know I have to. I push myself up and look over the seat and now can look into the rear seat next to the girl. There, strapped into his car seat and secured to the plane seat, is a smiling baby boy. One quick look at him and I don't think he seems to be injured.

Turning my attention back to the man in the middle seat, I place my fingers on his neck, feeling for a pulse, and indeed, he has one and is breathing. I then pinch him on the shoulder, and he lets out a moan. At that point, I decide that he is in as good a place as any and, stepping into the plane, ask the girl if she can help me get the car seat out. I want to pull the baby out and quickly check him before moving to the more complicated extrications of the girl and the two remaining men. With her good arm, she is able to unbuckle the car seat, and I am able to move the unconscious man enough to let Dennis in to help pull the car seat up and over the middle row of seats and take the infant out of the plane. I tell the girl I'll be right back, as I want to take a look at the toddler and let Bruce know what is going on and try to come up with a plan on how we are going to get all these people out of here.

Bruce has been able to safely remove the man from the wing and has him simply floating around it and has managed to bring him to the shore close to the area that we are now placing all our patients in. As we are discussing what our plan is going to be, we hear the distinct sound of rotor blades.

Looking up, we suddenly see the CHP helicopter fly over us and turn into a tight circle. Bruce, Dennis, and I quickly decide that Dennis should go back to the sandbar and inform the CHP crew that we will need their paramedic to help us and see if they can radio out to dispatch to have the sheriff's helicopter go to the staging area and load up with backboards and one of the ambulance crews. We will use the smaller sheriff's helicopter to simply shuttle men, women, and equipment into the scene. We will then use our helicopter and the CHP helicopter to transport the patients out.

Dennis nods in agreement, and as he turns to wade the river to meet up with the CHP crew, I yell at him to wait a minute. I reach down, and as I raise up the car seat with the infant in it, I hand it to him, telling him to just buckle him in one of the seats. We will fly him down and out of here with our first patient transport. Dennis grabs the loaded car seat with both hands and, raising it above his head, starts into the river. I turn back to Bruce and ask how his patient is. He tells me that he definitely has a spinal cord injury, that he has no feeling or movement from his waist down, but that he remembers the entire event. He told him that after they took off from the Paradise Airport, they were flying okay when the engine suddenly lost power. The pilot was able to baby it along, but with it fully loaded with six passengers, the single-engine aircraft just couldn't hold altitude. They started down the canyon as the pilot tried everything he could think of to keep it going, but it was obvious that they were going down. As the plane slammed into the embankment of the river, his door flew open and he suddenly found himself being torn from his seat and landed on the wing, trying to hold on for dear life.

We both look up and can see Dennis now returning with the two CHP officers, and as they wade across the river, they meet up with us. They have brought any and all equipment they have on their ship, and the five of us now discuss our plan. The CHP pilot and paramedic will stay and help get the unresponsive man from the middle seats and then the girl from the rear. I will start out with the unresponsive woman that is now lying on the embankment and return with more supplies. The CHP crew will fly out the unresponsive man from the middle seat, and maybe the girl, if they can fit her in their Long Ranger. Bruce will stay and continue with treatment and extrication until more help arrives with the sheriff's helicopter. We all agree that the pilot is going to be the last to be transported, as we can all see that he is really wedged between the seat and dash, and it will simply take a while to get him out, and at this point, we will wait for reinforcements to arrive.

All in agreement, we start out into our different directions. As Dennis and I place our woman onto a backboard, secure her, then start across the river, it is a real struggle. The water is deep at this point, and the last thing we want to do is slip and drop her. We finally make it to the other embankment and easily make it across the shallow part of the river and slide her into the A-Star. As I start securing her and attaching all the equipment, I take a quick look at our other passenger. Dennis has seat-belted the car seat into Bruce's seat, and surprisingly, the young infant is just looking up at me, smiling.

I decide the only real treatment this little one is going to need is just some words of encouragement. So as I'm starting IVs and intubating the woman, I give a verbal description of what I'm doing, looking at the infant for approval. "So is this your mommy? Is it okay if I start an IV on her? Do you want to help me tape it down?" I intermittently look at him, and he keeps smiling, as if he is approving everything I'm doing, then as the rotor blades start turning, he is distracted from my duties and is mesmerized by the spinning of the rotors.

In no time, Dennis has the turbine up to full power and pulls up on the collective, and the A-Star lifts from the sandbar. I take a quick look out the window and can see not only the remaining two crews working at the crash but also the CHP helicopter sitting on the sandbar just behind where we are. Knowing the sheriff's helicopter will more than likely be there when we return, I make a mental note to take a picture of the scene when we return.

Being alone in the helicopter is making the work twice as hard as having a partner. Add to that that I actually have two passengers, even though all I'm doing is smiling and talking to the youngster. I have attached the ventilator to the ET tube I have placed in the woman to free myself up and have been able to start two IVs and attach the woman to the pulse oximeter and cardiac monitor. A quick look out the window and I can see that Dennis is already banking the helicopter around for an approach to the helipad. I suddenly remember I forgot to call a report to the hospital. Dennis has kept them up to date on our ETA, but I'm sure the trauma team is wondering what I'm dropping off. At this point, it is too late; we are touching down and the unloading crew is approaching. I decide that I should have a little time after we lift off and the team is taking the patient down in the elevator to still call in a report and have it done before the patient rolls into the trauma room.

I quickly slide the door open and detach all the monitoring equipment. The woman is out in seconds, and the crew takes over, assisting her ventilations. I then climb back into the running helicopter and unbuckle the car seat and gently step out with the baby. As I look at him, he is at first looking at me with a big smile as I tell him, "You take care, pal. I'll check on you in a while." I then hand the entire package to one of the ED techs. Our techs are usually young college students, which also means most of them aren't married yet, don't have children of their own, and holding an infant scares the hell out of them. I can also see that he is being very careful, maybe overly cautious.

I yell into the ear of the nurse that I will radio in a report to the trauma team as soon as we take off. She nods, and I bend over, grabbing the second gurney that the techs have brought up and slide it into the ship. As I climb back into the helicopter, I buckle in and give Dennis a thumbs-up, and he lifts the helicopter off the pad and we start our trip back to the crash scene. As I'm trying to organize the equipment inside, I decide to not close the door; it is really hot out, and we will be on scene in roughly ten minutes, and the air-conditioning will not have much effect in that short amount of time. The air flowing through the cabin feels good and is helping cool us off a little.

I have things back together just as we are clearing the ridge and starting our descent back to the sandbar. Dennis has filled me in that the sheriff's helicopter has made two trips in carrying in some ambulance crew, backboards, and light extrication equipment to help us get everyone out. As we are now banking around the trees and I can see the two other helicopters sitting on the sandbar, with the different EMS workers doing different tasks around the wreckage of the plane, with its one wing in the water, I suddenly remember I wanted to take a picture of the scene, and looking out, I now know this might be a Pulitzer Prize–winning photo and remember I've forgotten my camera today but know there should be a camera kept in the helicopter. I quickly grab the hospital's camera out from under the bench seat where it is kept. I know I will have to take a moment to jump out of the helicopter after we land and get behind it to get it in the scene with all three helicopters sitting on the sandbar and the wrecked plane in front of all of them.

As I'm getting excited about my once-in-a-lifetime shot, I'm looking out the open door, trying to spot where I should take the photo from to have all three helicopters, the crashed plane, and all the workers in view, when Dennis starts banking into the final landing approach. Suddenly, I feel something hit my leg. I look down, and as if time has turned into slow motion, I can see all four of the double-A batteries sliding out of the camera and exiting the aircraft through the open door.

"NOOOOOOO!" I yell as I put my head out the door and watch as the tiny batteries drift through the air and make small splashes as they hit the water.

Dennis, being a little concerned as to what I'm yelling about, quickly asks, "What's up?"

I hold up the camera with the small battery door open, and he laughs.

"No way! Did they really just fall out?"

"Yes. Can you believe that? There goes my chance at the cover shot for the *Air Medical Journal*."

Totally mad at myself that I've let this happen, I fight back the urge to just toss the entire camera out the door and into the lake.

Dennis is still laughing as he is setting the ship down on the sand, and as if not to let it just go, he has to get the last word. He turns, looking at me, and, with a huge smile, says, "Well, I guess you had better not quit your day job."

"Very funny," I answer as I'm stepping out of the ship and pulling off my helmet.

I grab the fresh first-out bag that the unloading crew has brought up to me with the second gurney and start out across the water and make my way back to the crash site. As I'm wading through the deep water and approaching the plane, I can see the CHP officers have a patient loaded up and are about to make the trip to their helicopter. "Where do you want me?" I ask out load, primarily addressing my partner, who I'm sure is running things, as he has been here the longest.

Bruce takes a quick look at me and then directs me to help the CHP officers carrying their patient across the water and load him into their helicopter. I nod and turn my attention to the officers and ask, "What do you need me to do?" They instruct me that they just want help carrying and crossing the water. "No problem," I answer, and before grabbing one end of the backboard that the patient is secured to, I toss the first-out bag onto the shore. I also see that one of their packs is lying close to me. I reach down, grab it, and sling it over my shoulders, then lift my end of the board. Looking down, I can make out the face of the man that has been unresponsive in the middle seat, whom I've had to lean over to assess the girl and infant in the rear seats. The three of us then make the trip across the deep water, almost holding the patient over our heads before lowering him down as we reach the other side. We walk down the far embankment and then wade the shallow water and reach the Bell helicopter. The paramedic then instructs me that since I have the foot end, I need to start that end in first, then we will slide the patient in the rest of the way. The pilot then starts securing the board to the ship as the paramedic starts attaching equipment. I hold the IVs up as this is happening and can spot a hook on the ceiling that I'm assuming I can attach the IVs to. Now setting the backpack onto the floor, the paramedic turns and thanks me for helping. Stepping away, I give him a thumbs-up as I tell him, "See you soon." Knowing they will be making a return trip.

I make my way back across the river, and as I'm climbing out onto the embankment, I check in with Bruce. I can see that he has all the other firefighters and EMS crew that the sheriff has flown in hard at work. The ambulance EMT and paramedics are taking care of all the passengers that have all been removed from the airplane and are laying on backboards on the shoreline, and it appears that the firefighters are involved in beating the airplane apart to get the pilot out. Bruce is standing next to the plane, watching this, and as I walk up to him, I ask, "What's up?"

Without turning to look at me, he starts telling me, "I think they are going to have him out very soon, and we should fly him out next."

"Okay," I answer, now trying to concentrate more on what is going on with this patient, then ask, "Are you going to fly him, or do you want me to take him?"

"I want you to take him," he starts, then finishes his explanation as we take a few steps away from the plane, looking back at all the remaining patients on the shoreline. "I pretty much know what is going on here and have somewhat of a plan. I think it would be too hard to hand all this off, so if you don't mind, go ahead and start in on the pilot. I'll get the CHP to take one or two more, then when you return, we should be able to take the final patient."

Nodding, I have to agree that this sounds like a good plan and can see that he has thought this through. "Okay, I'll grab my bag and start in with him." As I point at the pilot. Bruce and I nod at each other then turn and go our separate ways. As I approach the front of the airplane, I can see one of the firefighters must be the captain, as he is wearing a red helmet. Walking up to him, I ask, "Hey, do you think you'll have him out soon?"

The captain steps back to talk with me as his two firefighters continue with what they are doing. "You know," he starts in, then hesitates, "I think we will have him out in just a few minutes."

I then ask if anyone has done an exam on him, and just looking from where I am, I can tell he is somewhat slumped over the steering column and moaning. Someone has placed him on oxygen, but I don't see any IVs running.

"Not really. We could only get to his upper torso. He will open his eyes if we inflict some pain, but he really isn't talking at all, only moaning."

That's pretty much what I've figured from my vantage point. I then ask if I can take a few seconds to do a quick exam. He nods, then tells his crew to step aside for a moment.

I crawl into the airplane through what used to be the door, and as I kneel in the passenger seat, I start asking the patient questions to see if he will answer me at all. "Hey, buddy, what's your name?" He doesn't answer, and I repeat the question as I now pinch him fairly hard on his shoulder. "Hey, buddy, what's your name?" He only moans and shrugs his shoulder, telling me that he more than likely has a head injury. I then take my stethoscope and listen to his chest. As I move the diaphragm into different locations, it is very apparent that he has no lung sounds on his right side. Removing my stethoscope, I palpate his chest and can instantly feel the grinding of broken ribs on the right side of his chest. Knowing that he has a collapsed lung, and possibly a tension pneumothorax, I continue with what assessment I can complete. It looks as if both of his forearms are broken, as I'm betting he had a death grip on the yoke when the plane hit, snapping both of his wrists. I can't really tell much about his abdomen with him still in the sitting position, and the same about his pelvis. I attempt to check out his legs but can only run my hands down to about his knees. Pulling my hands back, I'm thinking of all the things that need to be done to this guy, IVs, possibly intubate him, possibly decompress a tension pneumothorax, let alone all the splinting. I back out of the plane and motion for the firefighters to continue with the extrication as I talk to the captain.

"He really isn't doing well," I start, then continue with part of my plan. "I'd really like to start an IV on him now to replace some of the fluid he has lost, if you don't mind?"

The captain nods, telling me that would be fine. I reassure him that I can do this while staying out of their way. In agreement, I flood an IV of normal saline and grab the necessary equipment I will need. The firefighters have already removed most of the seats from the plane and are now trying to get his either unlocked or loosened from the floor so they can slide him back away from the dash and engine. I walk around to the opposite side of the plane, and knowing the window is broken out, as I'm standing on the wing, I am able to pull the patient's left arm out through the window and start an IV in the upper part of his arm without much problem. I open up the clamp and let the solution run in as fast as it can, giving him a bolus. After laying the bag on top of the airplane to free up my hands, I attempt to splint the forearm that is severely broken. Wrapping it up, I then slide the arm back into the aircraft just as the firefighters say they are now ready to see if the seat is going to move. I jog back around the aircraft and, picking up a backboard along the way, wait outside as I watch the three firefighters shake the chair loose from its attachment on the floor. It suddenly pops loose, and instantly, the seat and patient start to lie down backward. The fire crew then slowly work the seat back until the patient is away from the mangled dash. From my vantage point, I spot a solution to getting him out maybe a little easier and speak up with a possible plan. "Hey, wait a minute." The firefighters stop what they are doing and look at me. "Why don't we just leave him in that seat and bring him out of the plane in it, then we will move him onto a backboard out here? I think that would not only be easier but also quicker. What do you think?" The firefighters, all nodding now, looking at the cramped quarters they are in, can see this might work really well.

The captain then steps out of the plane, and when he is out on the wing, the two of us reach down and the two firefighters left inside the plane lean the seat back to us. We grab the top of the seat and, with the two inside lifting the bottom, simply slide the pilot out of the aircraft and carry him and the seat all in one package over to a space on the embankment where we can safely move him over to the backboard. We gently set the seat down in a reclined position and prepare the patient to transfer him over. One of the firefighters grabs the board, one is releasing him from his harness, and I'm cutting away his clothing. All four of us then gently lift him out of his seat and place him onto the backboard, leaving his clothing behind.

I am now able to finally complete my assessment as the fire crew straps him down to the board. His left femur is fractured, and I believe his right ankle is broken. Knowing that our traction splint is still in the helicopter, I tell the firefighters that I just want to get him over to the ship now and we will put a traction splint on before we load him in. I then reassess his chest one last time before we lift to move him, still worried about the collapsed lung. It still doesn't sound good, and I can see his respirations have increased. I then tell the firefighters, "Let's go!" motioning for them to pick him up.

We start our trip across the river, and as we are working down the embankment, I can hear the CHP helicopter making its return approach to the sandbar. "Shit!" I say out loud as I'm looking at the landing zone, knowing that we are going to have to stop and let them land before making the last crossing to our helicopter. We kneel down and set our patient on the ground, and I wave for the approaching helicopter to land.

The Bell Long Ranger is making its distinctive *whop, whop, whop* of the two-blade rotor system as it pulls a lot of power before setting down onto the sand. As we are going to have to walk past the still-running helicopter, I wave to the crew a hand signal that we would like to continue toward our ship. The CHP paramedic has stepped out and waves us by. The firefighters and I then pick up our patient once again, and we continue stepping down into the water, then up onto the sandbar. As we are passing the running helicopter, the paramedic asks if this patient is for them. I yell at him over the noise of the blades and turbine engine, "No! I'll be taking this patient, but Bruce already has another patient waiting for you!" He nods, and as he turns back to the pilot to fill him in, we continue to the waiting A-Star.

We slide the patient into the ship with the assistance of Dennis, who has been helping the sheriff unload some equipment that he has flown in. Now with the patient secured, I'm buckled in, and the door closed, I recheck my patient, whose airway I have been worried about. Knowing that I may have to intubate him, I decide to try an oral airway first to see if he tolerates it. If so, I'll place the ET tube. I pull the oral airway out of the bag and slide it into the patient's mouth; to my surprise, he doesn't gag, cough, or even flinch.

"Dang!"

"What dang?" Dennis asks.

I look up at him briefly before reaching for the intubation equipment. "I'm going to have to intubate him," I tell him, then ask, "What's our ETA?"

Looking down at the GPS on the dash, he then answers back, "About five minutes."

"Shit, okay, I think I can get this done in five minutes."

Now knowing I have a challenge to meet, I quickly pull the tube out, lubricate, place the stylet, check the cuff with the attached syringe, then place it on the patient's chest as I reach in the bag and pull out the laryngoscope handle and select the blade size I think will work the best. I then pull the oral airway out and, almost in the same maneuver, slide the blade down into the patient's mouth and visualize as it slides down the back of his throat until I see his vocal cords. I reach up with my other hand and grab the prepared ET tube and quickly slide it into position. I can feel as the balloon at the end is making its slight vibration as it passes through the vocal cords. Quickly I pull out the blade then the stylet out of the tube. As I air up the cuff, I can see some condensation forming in the tube, which gives me a pretty good idea that the tube is in the correct place. To double-check, and because the patient is still breathing, I can hold my hand over the end of the tube and feel his exhalation as he breathes through the tube. I don't feel I have to assist his respirations with a bag valve device and just place the nonrebreather mask over the end of the tube. I look up at the monitor, and I can see that his oxygen saturation is in the high nineties, and I tape the tube to the patient's face. Now I know if he should vomit, his airway is protected.

After I tear the last piece of tape securing the tube to his face, I take a quick look out the window and I can see we are only a minute out from the hospital. "I guess I should call in a report," I tell Dennis as he is starting to bank the helicopter into the final approach at the helipad.

"You had better hurry!" he says with a little chuckle in his voice.

I manage a smile as I reach down and press the transmit button on the cord to my helmet. "Enloe Hospital, FlightCare, med channel 8, ETA one minute!"

The base nurse must have been waiting for me, as she instantly answers me, "FlightCare, Enloe Hospital, copy ETA one minute. Go ahead!"

"On final approach with a thirty- to thirty-five-year-old male who was the pilot of the airplane. He was most certainly trapped in the aircraft for some time, pinned between the seat and the dash. He has a decreased LOC, withdrawing from pain and moaning. Pupils are equal, his airway was questionable and has been intubated. Decreased lung sounds on the right with crepitus to the right thorax. Abdomen is soft and flat, pelvis appears intact. I see bilateral fractures of his arms and a left femur fracture. He is breathing on his own, and I have O_2 by blow-by at 15 liters per minute. Pulse ox is 97 percent. His vital signs are as follows." Now looking up at the monitor to read off the findings, I continue, "Blood pressure is 110 over 72, pulse is 98." Turning to look out the window, I suddenly feel the skids coming into contact with the helipad. I finish with, "And we're here!"

I release the transmission button and reach down and unlock then slide the door open. The receiving crew, crouching over, approaches the running helicopter in what is becoming a well-rehearsed rhythm for them today. We quickly slide our patient out, and as the nurse takes over, I yell a couple of comments to her so she knows to watch the airway. I don't want our patient to suddenly reach up and pull the tube out of his lungs. She nods, then turns to start down the ramp. The ED tech is already sliding the other gurney into the ship, and as he hands me the first-out bag, he tells me that he really hasn't had time to restock it for me but has thrown a couple of IV sets into it. I thank him, toss it onto the gurney, and climb back in. I have not removed my helmet and have not even unplugged the cord, so all I have to do is buckle in. Dennis already has the RPMs at full speed, and as I feel the last buckle click, I tell him one word, "Buckled!" Immediately he is pulling up on the cyclic, and the helicopter, now with much less fuel and short one crew member, jumps off the helipad.

I decide to not close the door once again for the ten-minute flight back to the lake. With very little conversation, I try to organize the inside, and I can tell that I'm running out of room to store all the garbage. I then remember the drawer under the jump seat. I slide the drawer open and start stuffing it full of empty IVs, tubing wrappers, dirty laryngoscopes, and all the miscellaneous wrappings of different bandages. With a final push from both my hand and right foot, I get the drawer closed. Jokingly, I tell Dennis to not let me forget to clean it out or day shift will shit a brick when they find it full of trash.

Just as I sit back into my seat, I can hear Dennis talking to the CHP helicopter. He then asks me to help him look for it, as it is already en route with a patient and heading directly toward us. We both strain, looking out the front windshield when the two of us spot the Bell helicopter at the same time, with both of us yelling, "There it is!" Dennis makes a small adjustment in our flight, banking a little to the right, and, at the same time, keys the microphone, telling the CHP crew that we have a visual on them and will be passing them on their left. The CHP pilot acknowledges, and within a minute, the two of us pass in opposite directions. I still have the door open and manage a wave as we pass.

Sitting back and relaxing for a minute, I am taking stock on what we have done and what may be left to do when I ask Dennis, "I think there should only be one patient left there, the girl from the rear seat." Dennis agrees with me, then we start talking about the remaining fire and ambulance personnel that will be left there but both agree the sheriff's helicopter has brought them in and will more than likely be flying them out. As we are finishing our conversation, Dennis is banking the A-Star over and making the final approach to the sandbar. Just before setting down, I look up at the plane and can see that the young girl is already strapped to a board, and it looks as if they are about to start carrying her across the river, making the trip to us. I inform Dennis what I think is going on, that maybe after landing, he should keep the ship running, adding, "I'll jump out, and if they are indeed bringing her to us, we can just load her up and leave." As he sets the ship down onto the sand, he agrees, and unplugging my helmet but leaving it on, I release my seat belt and hop out. As I start across the shallow water to the embankment, I can see the firefighters and Bruce wading across the deep water, and soon I meet up with them. I ask Bruce if this is the last patient, and he says yes. As we continue toward the running helicopter, I ask him if he is coming with us this time and if we will be returning.

He tells me, "Yes, we are done here, and there is no reason for us to return. The sheriff's helicopter will stay and remove all the first responders and the firefighters."

"Excellent," I answer him as we are now at the side of our helicopter and sliding the young girl into position. Bruce climbs in, and as I thank the firefighters for all their assistance, they smile and make their way back to the crashed plane. Buckled in, Dennis pulls up on the collective and we lift from the sandbar for the last time. After sliding the door closed, I start helping Bruce connect the different monitors to our patient.

As I take one last look out the window to see what our ETA is back to Enloe, I can see that the sun is now setting over the mountains to the west. Dennis swings the ship into a final approach to the helipad, and we can see that the CHP Long Ranger is still on the helipad, but they have set down off to the side so we could also land next to them. As we touch down, the ground crew approaches the helicopter, and I can hear Dennis telling me that he will be going to the airport for fuel. I unplug my helmet and help slide our young girl out of the ship onto the gurney and start our trip down the ramp and into the elevator. As we make our descent to the first floor, a wave of exhaustion suddenly comes over me. We have been nonstop for hours. I fight the feeling off as I know that in reality, I'm just starting my shift and there is still a long way to go.

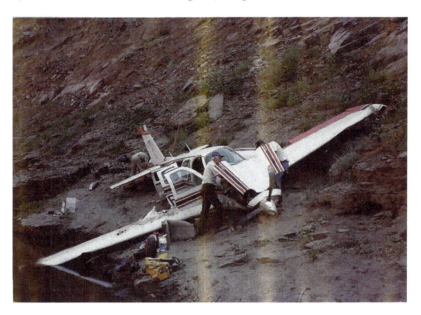

The elevator doors open, and as we walk into the ED, the charge nurse directs us to one of the treatment rooms to place the girl. As we walk by the trauma room, I can see a room full of people and hear the excitement of the room of either one of the prior patients I have brought in or one of the patients the CHP has brought in. We transfer our girl to one of the beds and report off to the nurse. As Bruce and I start wiping off the flight gurney, I look up at him and ask, "Do you have any idea what equipment we need?"

"I was hoping you kept track," he says with a smile.

About then, the two CHP officers walk up to us, and the paramedic says, "Wow, that was quite a disaster!"

"Yes, it was, and thanks for helping out. If you hadn't shown up, we would still be making trips back and forth."

We all chuckle a little, then the four of us talk a little about the scene and what we think had gone right and what we would do differently in the future. All the time, Bruce and I are pulling different equipment we think we will need to restock the helicopter. With our now two gurneys and two different first-out bags piled high with different bandages, IVs, oxygen equipment, and cleaning items, the four of us start down the hall to the elevator and start our trip up to the helipad.

Just as we exit the elevator, we hear the A-Star approaching and take our time walking up the ramp to give Dennis time to set down without blowing all our restocks off the roof. As we roll out onto the helipad, Dennis shuts down the engine and exits the ship. As Bruce and I start in with pulling out everything from inside and tossing it onto the helipad, the two CHP officers are joining in, helping with what they can do. All of us are talking about the call, the different patients, and the difficulty of managing such a call.

After we finish putting FlightCare back together, we carry our cleaning supplies over to the CHP helicopter and help them clean it out. We finally finish cleaning the two helicopters, and after a few handshakes, we say our goodbyes and watch as the Bell Long Ranger cranks up and lifts off into the night sky.

The three of us make our way down the elevator and back to the ED. We toss the trash into the biohazard container in the trauma room, knowing we have a mound of paperwork waiting for us. As Dennis heads back to the pilot's quarters, Bruce and I start searching out the different staff members that have helped take care of our patients, so we can get a report on them and obtain some information to complete our run reports. After gathering a mound of paper, we are both finally able to go to the computers and start our novels. It feels good to finally sit and relax, and I take a moment to just lean back and stretch.

As I am leaning back and have my arms outreached, I suddenly feel someone behind me grabbing my arms. I tilt my head almost over backward, and there, looking upside down, is Drena. She pulls my arms around her waist, and I pull her in, giving her a squeeze. She then lets go of my arms and wraps her arms around my neck, bending over and returning the hug, saying, "You've been busy."

About then, Bruce, watching us, speaks up, a little jealous. "Hey, where is my hug?"

Drena smiles, and I answer by telling him, "Find your own. This one is taken."

As the conversation continues between the three of us, Drena and I won't let go of each other. We laugh and talk about the call when Drena's pager starts beeping. Knowing she will have to leave, I give her one last squeeze before letting go and sitting up straight in my chair. She looks at her pager and tells us that one of our patients is coming out of surgery. She'll go check on them and try to catch the two of us later. She gives me one more squeeze around the neck then disappears around the corner.

As I turn my head from watching her walking away and back to the computer, I find Bruce staring at me when I finally have to ask, "What?"

He then asks, "When are you going to marry that girl?"

"I'm not sure," I answer, then add, "We have such a good thing, and we really enjoy each other's company. It isn't like we haven't talked about it. We both have busy careers, and we're not sure how it would all work out."

Without hesitating, Bruce, who has been happily married for well over ten years, tells me, "Well, I think the two of you were made for each other. You should just go do it and not worry about how it will work out."

"Yes, you're probably right."

Our conversation is interrupted by the ED charge nurse, who pops his head around the corner. "Hey, can one of you come help out? We are getting hammered."

Bruce speaks up first, saying he will go help. Since I flew most of the patients, I should stay and finish the reports. I agree, and as the two of them disappear around the corner, I reminisce about the call, all the patients we treated, and then spend the remainder of my time thinking about my friend Drena. She is stunningly beautiful, incredibly intelligent, and more loving than anyone I have ever met. Not just to the patients and the family members she has never met before their time at Enloe, but to everyone she meets.

 What will I do?

5

LONG NIGHT IN BI-COUNTY

WE ARRIVE AT work just before 1800 hours. The day crew is always thankful for us not being late, as they really want to get out of here on time. Most of them are family people; they have kids to pick up, dinner to prepare, and a glass of wine or a beer calling their name. The last thing they really want to do is to get dispatched on a flight to pick a patient up in Quincy to take to UC–Davis, which could take around three to four hours.

I am not a big believer in double standards. One rule for everyone! *Yeah, right*. Rarely is the receptacle effort of the day crew showing up early ever done for the night shift. I don't know how many times my boss has met with me, holding my time card in her hand, wanting to know why I have so much overtime or double time. A quick glance at the times will answer her question.

"Well, it's like this. We were dispatched on a long interfacility transfer at six fifteen in the morning," I say, staring at the time card.

Already knowing her next question, I still wait for her to ask, "Why were you leaving on a flight fifteen minutes after you got off work?"

Smiling, I answer, "It's simple, either I go with the ship and do the transfer or we put the helicopter out of service until the day relief shows up."

My answer is a little on the verge of being a smart-ass, but we have had this discussion multiple times in the past, and it is always the same answer. There are a couple of day shift crew that simply cannot get here on time. It also makes me mad and frustrated, as I always seem to be the one who gets the brunt of it. Then I ask, "Why don't you talk to them and tell them to be here on time? We don't care if they are a little early, but they definitely shouldn't be late."

She knows I'm right. She then tells me she will investigate with the day shift and tell them to be a little more responsible. I mention to her to also pass along that it costs the hospital overtime and double time when this happens. Let alone I don't like getting my butt chewed out for doing *their* job. She agrees and offers a hug to cool me off and lets me know that she really does care and she is just doing her job. We smile and joke a little when we are interrupted by the pager going off.

"FlightCare, scene flight near Strawberry Valley. Heading one nine eight degrees, thirty-five miles."

I pick up my bag and say goodbye to the boss as I exit the office. Looking down the hall, I can see my night partners already at the elevator, so I break into a jog to join up with them just as the elevator doors are opening. "Any idea what we are getting into?" I ask. There is no answer, as the nurse is putting the key into the slot in the elevator to give us an express ride to the roof. I look at Tom, our pilot, and he has a wide smile and shit-eating grin on his face, looking like the cat that has just eaten the canary. I can tell he wants to say something but is hesitant. Finally, as we are passing through the third floor, I ask, "What?"

Tom starts laughing and, through his laughter, finally gets out, "So what did you get your butt chewed out for this time?"

I look up, and the nurse is also laughing. "Those darn day-shifters," I start. "They show up late, I take the flight, then I get in trouble for double time." I am shaking my head in frustration as the elevator stops and the doors open in the ready room on the roof. We each grab our helmets, then jog up to the helipad. Nobody is giving me much of a break. They keep rubbing it in all the way up until we are fastening our seat belts and pulling on our helmets. About that time, dispatch is calling us to give us more details, for which I am thankful, as I really want to get off this subject.

"Go ahead, dispatch," I transmit as Tom is cranking the turbine. Dispatch comes back on, giving us our rendezvous location and ground contact information. They then tell us that even though this is reported as a cardiac patient, they think this may be up a canyon in a remote spot, possibly a hiker. As I acknowledge, I can see that we are lifting from the helipad, and I finish my transmission with, "Copy that, and FlightCare is on the go!"

As I slide my door closed, we pull out a map of the area to try to get an idea where we may be headed. It looks to be out of Strawberry Valley, possibly up Strawberry Canyon, and it should take us about twenty to twenty-five minutes to arrive over the scene.

Cruising along, we think we are about halfway there as we are inputting the frequencies into the radio when dispatch calls us. "FlightCare, per the Plumas County Sheriff's Office, you can cancel." We look up from the radio, and Tom starts a slow bank to the left, and I key up the radio. "Copy that, dispatch. FlightCare is canceling."

As we sit back in our seats, I reach down and pull the 2" tape off my thigh of my flight suit that I have been writing the contact information on, wad it up, and only momentarily discuss why we think we got canceled. Was the ambulance able to transport without us? Did the patient refuse to go by helicopter? Or did the patient die? In reality, we will probably never know, and because of this, we quickly get off the subject and start giving Bruce a hard time about a bachelor party he recently attended.

"Is it true what they say you did with one of those strippers?" I ask.

Before he has a chance to answer, Tom jumps in. "Man, what I heard you did borders on criminal. Matter of fact, I heard the SPCA is back at the ED, wanting to ask you some questions."

By now, Tom and I are laughing and Bruce is calling us names and telling us, "We don't need to be starting RUMORS about something that didn't happen."

Of course, I can't let it rest. We still have about a fifteen-minute ride to the airport, plenty of time to rub this in some more.

"Wait a minute," I ask, "you telling me this is all rumors?"

Bruce answers immediately as if we are really caring what he says, "Yes, those are rumors that someone started, and I don't want anything like that getting back to my wife." His demands are stern. I smile, looking out the window, knowing that with our intercom, I don't need to be looking at him to talk, as I wouldn't be able to keep a straight face, and continue, "You telling me you didn't go to the bachelor party?"

There is a short hesitation before he answers, "Well, yes, I did go."

Now I know I've got him, and I start in, "Okay, so you first told us all this was nothing but rumors and none of it was true, but now you are telling us that you actually were there!" I can feel the anxiety mounting and can see Tom is wiping tears from his eyes as he is entering Chico airspace, and I finish my question. "So that means the rumors must be true!" I say as I turn to look at him with a big smile on my face.

Bruce now knows there is no way out of this rough crowd and, after a moment, thinking through several answers, any of which would only make matters worse, simply says, "Screw you, guys!"

Tom and I are busting up. By the time we land at the airport for fuel, we are still prodding Bruce but also let him know that it is his turn to be the butt of all the joking. We would never do or say something that would get someone in trouble with their mate—well, almost never!

As we finish refueling the helicopter and are just starting to crank the engine, dispatch calls us on the radio and informs us that there is a patient to be picked up in Chester and taken to Redding Medical Center (RMC). "Cool," we all say in unison. This should take about four to five hours, successfully keeping us out of the ED for most of our shift.

As we are lifting from Chico and Tom is climbing and heading for the Chester Airport, I suddenly sit forward and yell into the intercom, "Shit, I forgot something!" Tom is looking over his shoulder at me as he is thinking I have forgotten to put the fuel cap back on or left an outside door open. Then he asks, "What?" I turn my head and look at Bruce, then key up the intercom. "I forgot the dude from the SPCA is waiting for you back in the ED." Bruce slugs me in the shoulder as Tom and I start laughing all over again.

The rest of the trip to Chester is full of conversation of Bruce trying to keep us off the bachelor party subject. By the time we set down at the Chester Airport, the hospital has contacted us and told us they need us to come into the hospital in the ambulance to pick up the patient. As Tom is shutting down the ship, Bruce and I are gathering all the items we think we will need. We know this is a medical patient that is having a heart attack and is to be transported to the cath lab at RMC. As we are strapping down the infusion pumps, we see the ambulance pulling onto the tarmac and wave it over to us. The EMT has come out by himself, leaving the paramedic back in the hospital. We know him and start with the usual greetings, leading to questions about the patient we are picking up.

He tells us that it is an elderly woman that they had gone out on earlier in the ambulance to pick up at her house and she was having chest pain. When they did a twelve-lead EKG back in the ER, it showed she was having an infarct. He then tells us that she actually lives in Redding and was only up here at her cabin for the weekend.

We know this is somewhat normal, and because I also work at one of the Lake Almanor Fire Departments, I know more than 50 percent of the homes here are just summer homes or weekend retreats. At our fire department, we will see the population change from approximately one thousand in the winter to over five thousand on the weekends in the summer.

We arrive at the hospital and, with the EMT's help, roll the gurney into the ER to find a lot of familiar faces anxious to great us. The doctor and the nursing staff are almost always the same. We all work together in receiving a report, changing all the IV medications over to our pumps, placing her onto our monitors, then asking her how she is doing and telling her about her helicopter ride. We explain we will also put a headset on her so she can talk to us and that it is really important to let us know if her chest pain is getting worse or if anything else happens to her. She smiles and tells us she understands as we are now pushing the gurney into the back of the ambulance. The one-mile ride to the waiting helicopter is over before we know it, and we put an extra blanket over her as we move her out to the helicopter.

The sun has set, and it is fairly cold now. I explain that as soon as we get the engine fired up, Tom will crank up some heat for her. I can tell she is a little anxious about the whole ordeal when Tom speaks up and asks her if she has ever flown in a helicopter before. "No, never," she says. Tom then takes a moment to talk to her as Bruce and I switch everything over from the portable equipment to the onboard. Tom is able to reassure her that she will be okay and to just sit back and enjoy the ride.

As the engine is now fired up and our headsets are on, I reach down and unplug the patient for a second and tell Tom, "Nice job. I think you calmed her down a little."

Before Tom can answer back, Bruce adds in, "Yeah, it is probably a good thing not to tell her about the three helicopters you crashed in Vietnam."

I start laughing, and after Tom chuckles for a moment, he answers back, "Yeah, probably not a good thing to tell her war stories and how we were just blown out of the sky."

We get all the infusion pumps set, O_2 running, pulse oximeter working, and the cardiac monitor monitoring. About fifteen minutes into our flight, there is little to no conversation. The patient is looking out the windows, and Bruce and I are pretty much doing the same thing. I am still thinking about the scene call to Strawberry Valley and wondering what it may have been all about when suddenly I am snapped out of my daze by multiple alarms flashing and loud buzzing.

At first, I am stunned and wonder, *What the hell?* Bruce is doing the same when I make out that it's the cardiac monitor alarming, and I can see the cardiac rhythm has changed from a normal sinus rhythm to ventricular fibrillation (V-fib). At first, I don't believe it, as it can also look this way if one of the monitor leads works loose off the patient. I gently reach down and shake the shoulder of our patient, asking, "Are you all right?" About then, Bruce turns the light on, and I can see in an instant that our patient has gone from smiling and pink to unresponsive and blue. "Shit!" I say as I am now reaching down to lower the head of the gurney and yell into the headset, "She has coded!"

Bruce can see what I'm doing and is already reaching for the defibrillator paddles as I am grabbing the Ambu bag to start breathing for her. I give her a couple of quick breaths, then reach down and make a cut through the front of her blouse with my scissors so Bruce can pull it apart and apply the paddles and administer a defibrillation to her heart.

"Clear!" Bruce yells into the intercom, followed almost immediately by pushing the buttons. The woman bounces off the gurney, then falls back into her same position. We both look at the monitor and see that she is still in V-fib. "Clear!" Bruce yells again, and again, the woman bounces first up, then down onto the gurney. This time, as we look at the monitor, we can see that her rhythm has changed back to a normal sinus rhythm. I reach down, placing two fingers onto her neck to feel for a carotid pulse, and, within a few seconds, announce, "She has a pulse."

Bruce and I both fall into different jobs that the two of us know so well. I continue to breathe for her, and he starts turning off all the infusion pumps and is pulling out some lidocaine to administer to hopefully stabilize her heart. "Are you going to intubate her?" Bruce asks as he is pushing the medication.

I pause for a moment, then tell him, "I think I'll bag her for a few minutes and see if she starts coming back around before putting a tube in."

Sure enough, within a couple of minutes, our patient is starting to moan and is moving around. I apply a nonrebreather oxygen mask, and as I'm trying to passively restrain her, I'm also trying to talk to her and reorient her, telling her that it is okay, that she is in a helicopter en route to the hospital in Redding. Bruce has pulled out a lidocaine drip and is trying to flood the tubing when I notice my flailing patient go limp again. A quick look up at the monitor and I know why. "She's back in V-fib!" I yell as I reach for the Ambu bag again with one hand and pull the oxygen mask from her face with the other.

"Shit!" Bruce says in frustration as he sets the IV drip down and grabs the defibrillation paddles once again. "Clear!" he yells, and for the third time, the woman's body leaps off the gurney and back.

ON THE GO

We both stare at the monitor, and sure enough, one, then a second normal heartbeat appears. I already have my fingers on her neck, and I let Bruce know that, once again, we have a heartbeat!

I start assisting her respirations once again, and Bruce once again reaches for more lidocaine. As he pushes it, I mention that although I know he is busy, we really need to get that IV infusion going to help keep her from going back into V-fib for a third time. "I know, I know!" he shouts as he is working feverishly. Tom speaks up and asks if there is anything he can do. "Yes," I start. "Contact RMC and tell them that the patient has coded twice. We currently have a rhythm, starting her on a lidocaine drip, and give our ETA."

"Okay," he says, then looks down at the console to change the radio channel to the EMS frequency.

Bruce has finally gotten the lidocaine running and is trying to adjust it, and I can hear Tom calling in the report to RMC, and he is also letting them know we will be there in about ten minutes.

This time, the woman isn't waking up as she did before, and I decide to go ahead and intubate her. Bruce hands me the tube and laryngoscope, and I am able to put the tube in quickly. I attach it to the Ambu bag and start looking at the monitor for what her oxygen saturation might be. Just as I notice that it is reading 97 percent, I notice the normal sinus rhythm start looking, not normal. At first, there are a few, then a lot of PVCs (premature ventricular contractions). I am midway through my sentence, telling Bruce what I see, when the PVCs turn to V-fib again. I don't have to say anything as I hear Bruce once again yelling, "Shit!" as he is reaching for the paddles.

"Clear!"

I barley have time to let go of the bag when the woman bounces off the gurney. We are both staring at the monitor, oblivious to anything else, when we suddenly feel the skids coming into contact with the rooftop. A quick glance out the window and I can see we have landed on the helipad and see the receiving team of about five or six people staring at us. As I slide the door open and wave them over, I can hear Bruce yelling once again, "Clear!" I let loose of the

Ambu bag, and the woman bounces up, then back. I grab the bag and squeeze a couple more breaths as we can see she is still in V-fib.

"Clear!" Bruce yells for a third time, and louder, as the team of nurses, ER techs, and the cardiologist have all arrived and are standing just outside the open door as I am holding a hand out, motioning for them to wait and not approach. Bruce pushes the buttons for the third time, and the woman once again bounces off the gurney. I grab the bag and squeeze with one hand and feel for a pulse with the other. I suddenly notice another pair of hands doing the same on the other side of her neck and assume this must be her physician.

"We have a pulse. Let's get her out of here and down to the cath lab, NOW!" he shouts.

I climb out of my seat, and it seems like only ten seconds and we have her out. I continue to breathe for her, while Bruce is holding the IVs and trying to keep the tubing from getting caught up. The ER tech is hooking up my Ambu bag to the oxygen on the gurney. The two nurses are trying to carry different items when the entire group enters the elevator. We are all squeezed into it. Bruce and I are still wearing our helmets, and even though I can see the physician's mouth moving and make out a few words, I can't understand what he is trying to ask me, so I motion for one of the nurses to take over with the bag so I can remove my helmet. The physician once again asks, "How many times have you shocked her?"

I think for a moment, then tell him, "Six, I think."

The words are barely out of my mouth when Bruce yells out, "She's in V-fib again!"

As Bruce is reaching for the paddles, the ER tech has jumped up on the side of the gurney and has started chest compressions. Just as the elevator doors open to a few stunned people, Bruce yells out, "Clear!" The tech stops compressions, I let go of the bag, and everyone steps back, including the people that are waiting for the elevator. The woman bounces off the gurney as Bruce delivers the shock, and before he is done, we are pulling the gurney out of the elevator and are walking at a very fast pace toward the cath lab. The people in the hallway don't have to be told to step aside, as everyone is using both arms and hands to do something as we push through the doors to the lab.

Normally, those of us not in surgical scrubs would stop at this point and pass off our patient to the cath crew, but that is not the case tonight. We all keep going, and when we enter the cath room, one of the nurses just pushes the cath table out of the way and we roll into its place. I am still assisting ventilations, while Bruce and the other nurses are trying to get the IVs straightened out and onto the hospital pumps. The cardiologist isn't waiting for any of us. He knows that he must get a catheter into this woman and up to her heart now if he wants to save her. From my vantage point at the head of the gurney, I watch as he skillfully places lines into her femoral artery and starts advancing the catheter. I look up on the video x-ray screen and watch as the end of the catheter gets closer to her heart. Soon the physician has it where he wants it and injects the dye. Instantly, he announces, "There it is!" We all stare at the screen and can see the totally occluded cardiac artery. The left anterior descending (LAD), otherwise known as *The Widow Maker*. This is the main artery that feeds blood to the largest part of the cardiac muscle.

The physician does a few magical things with his catheter, and within seconds, we can see that he has pushed through the occlusion and now the dye is passing through what is the blockage and to the remainder of the heart. "Got it!" he announces, and we all breathe a sigh of relief.

Our patient is now sedated by the anesthesiologist, who has come to our side and taken over for me, placing her onto a ventilator. Bruce and I finally find ourselves being replaced by the hospital staff and slowly escorted to the door of the lab. As we exit and watch the doors close behind us, we turn and stare at each other, then laugh. "Damn, that was exciting," I finally say. As we start walking back toward the elevator, we stop in front of it and look at each other, then almost simultaneously say, "Do you know where we are?" Once again, we start laughing. We have been to the ER and ICU many times, but neither of us has been to the cath lab before, and we really weren't paying attention on how we got there as we were working so hard on our patient.

We step into the elevator and start pushing buttons. "I can't even remember which level the ER is on," I say as I notice numbers that make little sense to us. RMC is in downtown Redding. Even though the ER is on the street level, I don't know what floor we are on, and the buttons in the elevator are of no help. There are only numbers, and they don't seem to take into account the basement. So I push all the buttons, and as the elevator starts moving up and opening on each floor, we stick our heads out, looking for anything that looks familiar. About the third time the doors open, a nurse dressed in scrubs enters. She must have thought we are crazy when we ask her which floor the ER is on.

We drop her off on the fourth floor and head back down to the second floor. Leaving the elevator, we start down the hallway, and soon we see signs and arrows pointing to the emergency department. When we enter, there are a couple of people we know that walk up to us, asking about our patient and wanting to know how our flight went. We tell them it was a real challenge and how she coded so many times but she did have a pulse when we dropped her off in the cath lab.

Soon we notice the ER tech, and I ask him if he could check with the cath lab and see if we can get our equipment back so we can leave. He walks over to a phone and makes a call. Soon he hangs up and tells us that they are done with it and will place it all on the gurney and push it outside the doors. Knowing the difficulty Bruce and I have just had finding the ER, we know we will never be able to find the cath lab, and I ask the tech if he wouldn't mind running down there and retrieving it for us. He smiles, knowing it is a maze, and agrees as he turns and starts out the ER doors into the abyss of the hospital.

The one thing I do know about this hospital is where the vending machines are, and I decide to make a run for a snack and a soda before we head out to the helicopter. I give Tom a quick call on the radio and ask if he wants anything, and he asks for the same, soda and chips. Bruce and I make our snack run, and as we are arriving back in the ER, we see the ER tech arriving with our gurney. We catch up and just keep pushing it to the elevator and ride up to the heliport. We arrive on the roof to find Tom is waiting there with some of the RMC LifeFlight crew and telling stories. We join in as we attempt to arrange our gurney and equipment back into some order before we take our seats and Tom starts up the turbine. A quick wave to the RMC crew and we are off the helipad, en route to the airport to take on some more fuel.

It is a quick trip, as I think it is less than a mile from the hospital. As the fuel guy is topping us off, the three of us are sipping sodas, munching on chips, and talking about our patient. Soon we are airborne again and headed back to Chico. By the time we set down on the rooftop at Enloe, I take a look at my watch and can't believe it is already one o'clock in the morning. We have been gone a total of seven hours. "I hope the ED isn't too busy," Bruce says as he is pulling off his helmet. We both know that one of us has to restock and the other has to start on the paperwork, and this report is going to be fairly complicated. "Yeah, me too" is all I say as I grab the dirty linen and the bag of trash from all the supplies we've used.

No such luck! As we enter the ED, we can see patients lined up in the hallway and everyone running around. As soon as the charge nurse sees us, she motions for us to approach her. Our arms are loaded with an assortment of used supplies, and she knows we have to get the ship back together but asks, "Can one of you help out here and the other go restock?" Bruce and I look at each other, and finally Bruce says, "Yeah, sure, I'll stay." He hands me his armload of used supplies and then pulls the paperwork and EKG rhythms from his pocket, and as he is setting them down on the top of my growing pile, the rhythm strips are literally in my face, and as he gives the papers one last push as if to Velcro them to my suit, he adds, "Maybe you could do the run report too." I can barely make out his face but do see his shit-eating grin.

"Yeah, fine!" I say in return. I slowly turn and start walking away and instantly can tell that I don't think I'm going to make it to the counter with all that is now overflowing from my arms. I can feel something sliding down my right side, and as I attempt to squeeze it with my elbow, I feel something else coming loose. I speed up in an attempt to make it to the counter before I lose everything, and as I make one last lunge, about half of my stuff comes loose and I literally toss everything toward the countertop, hoping that at least some of it will make it onto the counter and not the floor.

"Dang!" I say as I am now trying to catch more stuff by pressing my body up against the drawers, but to no avail; rhythm strips, face sheets, empty drug boxes, sheets, and defib wrappers are hitting the floor when I suddenly notice laughter behind me. As I turn, I see Drena walking up, laughing, and I ask, "You're not laughing at me, are you?"

"No, I would never laugh at you, but your twin is being really funny," she says as she helps push some of the stuff that is hanging over the edge up to the top of the counter.

As we both kneel down and start picking up some of the items I've lost onto the floor, she asks how our flight went. I start to tell her about the nice woman and then the events of her coding over and over and how we ended up in the cath lab. I suddenly notice a questioning look on her face and finally ask, "What?"

"I thought you went up some canyon to rescue someone?" she asks.

"Oh, yeah," I say, remembering that our original dispatch was for the Strawberry Valley incident. "We were canceled about halfway there and then were redispatched to Chester to take this woman to Redding."

"Boy, you've had a busy night," she says as we stand and pile up my lost items on the counter.

I then ask her if it has been this busy in the ED the whole time we were gone and tell her that the charge nurse has pulled Bruce to help in the ED and I have to restock the ship and do the paperwork. She tells me that yes, it has been very busy, but nothing really exciting, just the normal, humdrum stuff. She has no sooner finished her statement when her pager starts beeping and someone is calling her to the ICU. I tell her to have a good evening, and she does the same as she gives me a quick hug then turns and walks away down the hall.

By the time I've cleaned and put the ship together, sat, and finished my novel on our patient and attached all the different EKG rhythms, which, in itself, ends up to be five pages, it is close to five o'clock in the morning. I'm just breaking down the chart when the charge nurse walks around the corner to check on me and ask, "Have you eaten anything tonight?" I look up at her and tell her that I did have a small bag of chips and a soda at the airport in Redding. She then tells me that things are finally slowing down a little and to go ahead and grab something. I thank her, tossing my chart into the baskets, then head down to the cafeteria.

As I walk through the doors, I suddenly remember that they close at four o'clock for cleaning. I stand there for a moment and start thinking of the vending machines just outside the door when the cashier comes out with some cleaning wipes in her hands. "You need something?" she asks.

"I forgot you were closed," I tell her.

She then asks if I am looking for something special, and I tell her that no, I haven't eaten and am just looking for something to hold me over until I get home. "Wait a minute," she says as she sets her cleaning items down then disappears back into the kitchen. Within a minute, she reappears with a tin of apple pie with two slices left over in it and a scoop of ice cream on it. Handing it out to me, she asks, "Will this do?"

"Yeah!" I say with saliva building in my mouth.

I reach out with one hand and start unzipping my pocket for some money when she tells me, "Forget it. I was about to throw this stuff out. Just enjoy."

"Thanks!" I say with a smile.

I then grab a fork from the basket and take a seat. As the first bite of the dessert is melting in my mouth, I look around and notice that I'm the only one there. I decide to sit back, pull up another chair, and put my feet up and thoroughly enjoy my piece of pie.

"You call this work?" I suddenly hear from across the room.

I quickly put my feet back onto the floor, thinking some administrator has just walked in on me. It seems to never fail; you can be swamped all night, eleven out of twelve hours, saving lives, and the one moment when you sit down and pick up a newspaper or put your feet up to eat leftover apple pie, they will walk in. I turn in my chair and see Drena walking toward me, smiling.

"I was told you might be down here," she says as I offer her a chair next to me. I lean back and grab another fork from the basket and, without saying a word, offer it to her. She takes it, and for the next twenty minutes, we sit all alone in the cafeteria, sharing the pie and talking about our night.

After about thirty minutes, we have finished the pie and know we should be heading back to our own respective departments as the day shift will be coming in soon. We ride up the elevator together, stopping on the first floor to drop me off. As the doors open, I ask her if I'll see her again tonight. She says yes, that she'll be here. A quick hug and I step through the doors as they are closing, turning quickly to wish her a good day just as the doors close together.

I walk down to the ED and find the day crew just walking into the lounge, asking, "How was your night?"

"Just fine," I reply as I open my locker and grab my gear. Setting the keys and radio down on the table, I then finish my report "We went out twice, once toward Strawberry Valley, but were canceled, then a transfer from Chester to Redding, which got really exciting." I spend a little time telling them about the woman and how she coded so many times and how we had to remain with her all the way into the cath lab. About then, Bruce walks in and catches the end of our conversation, then adds, "Yeah, had to double-check my shorts after that one!" We all laugh, then we say our goodbyes. Bruce and I walk out together to the parking lot before climbing into our own cars and heading out in our different directions. By the time I reach my apartment, I can tell I'm exhausted. I walk in, feed my goldfish, a take quick shower, and before I know it, I'm out cold in my bed.

It seems to only have been ten minutes when I awake to the alarm. "No way!" I say as I reach for the alarm, double-checking the time. Two o'clock. "Shit!" I hold the clock on my chest as I fall back on my bed in defiance of what the clock is telling me. I slowly sit up then turn and let my feet drop to the floor. Rubbing my eyes, I look at the clock again as I set it back down on the nightstand. For a moment, I stare at the nightstand with the clock and lamp sitting on it and wonder, *If you work nights, shouldn't this be called a day-stand?* I chuckle to myself as I slowly put on my running clothes. By the time I get to the door, I'm more awake and grab my backpack with my gym clothes in it. Step outside, lock the door, put the key in the backpack, and start jogging to the gym. It is a typical summer afternoon in Chico—hot!

After the three-mile run to the gym, working out for an hour, then repeating the three miles back to the apartment, I grab a cold drink from the fridge and jump into the shower. It is a nice evening, so I decide to ride my bike to work. I strap my bag onto the back, double-check the light for the trip home, and soon I'm taking the back roads to the hospital, trying to avoid the main streets, as the traffic can be busy at this time, as most normal people are headed home. As I arrive at the hospital, I ride up onto the ambulance dock and dismount the bike, then lock it to the railing. I take the seat off and will put it and my helmet in my locker for safekeeping until the trip home in the morning.

The day crew has seen me come in, and they are working their way back to the lounge and enter just as Bruce comes in. "How was your day?" he asks.

"Boring," the day nurse says. "We went up, checked the ship, helped the mechanic wash it, then pretty much broke the ED nurses for breakfast and lunch breaks."

"Man, I don't know how all you day-shift people eat so much," I start, then add, "Whenever I do a day shift, it seems like all you do is eat. First, there is breakfast, then before you know it, lunch, then shortly after that, a break. When do you have time to take care of patients?" I am starting to get some looks from the day crew that I know all too well, and that look is to shut up and change the subject. "So you didn't go anywhere?" I ask as I reach for the keys and radio they have set on the table.

"No!" she says, and I can tell that was maybe a poor choice of a subject to change to, as now her x-ray eyes are staring inside of me, and I can tell she wants to reach in and pull out some vital organ when her death look and the conversation is suddenly broken with the beeping of a page on the radio. At first, we don't expect much. All of us thinking it is just our 18:00 evening pager test.

LONG NIGHT IN BI-COUNTY

"Enloe FlightCare, scene flight, Strawberry Valley, heading one nine eight degrees, distance thirty-five miles."

"Unbelievable!" the day crew says in unison. "I don't even know if we received a pager test today, and now you aren't here two minutes and you get a call."

Bruce and I can see the frustration on their faces and know the best recourse for us is to leave, now. Bruce grabs his keys and the radios off the table, and both of us bolt out of the room and head for the elevator, trying to restrain our laughter until we are at least out of range of anything being thrown at us. As we are standing at the elevator, waiting for Tom to run across the street, the two of us start laughing at first, then Bruce asks, "Isn't this exactly how last night started?"

"Yup, I believe so. You don't think we are being called back to the exact spot and same call as last night, do you?" In my mind, I am quite certain that this must be a different call, just by chance in the same location. I have had that happen before; it is rare, but possible. Then I think to myself, *Yeah, why would someone still be there at the same call for twenty-four hours?* No, not possible.

Tom has arrived, and the three of us are discussing the possibilities of having a call in the same place and giving some examples of the same that each of us has had. I bring up the fact that I know I have flown to Highway 70 and Woodruff Lane in Yuba County many times. Bruce tells us that he has been to a bad intersection near the Woodson Bridge in Tehama County multiple times. Then Tom breaks in, telling us, "Maybe we should avoid any place that starts with Wood." We all laugh as we are now leaving the heliport.

We radio dispatch that we are on the go, and they start giving us the latitude, longitude, radio frequency, contact name, and a brief description of the patient. A cardiac patient that was hiking and started having chest pain. We all look at one another and know that we are all having the heebie-jeebies. "Correct me if I'm wrong, but isn't that the exact same information and description of the patient we were sent for last night?" I ask.

"Yeah," Tom answers, looking down at the GPS, "that is also the exact same coordinates and frequency."

"All we need now is to be canceled," Bruce says, then ads, "at that point, I think we need to accept the realization that we may be in some episode of *The Twilight Zone!*"

We laugh, but in the back of my mind, I'm thinking, *You know, I think they had an episode like this. The same guy would wake up each morning and relive the same day. He was stuck in some time warp or something.*

Soon we have passed the point where we were canceled last night and know we are now flying into uncharted territory. From this point on, it is all new, and in reality, we feel better knowing that we aren't stuck in the same day forever. As we fly over the last ridge top and start descending into a canyon several miles north of the town of Strawberry Valley, we make contact with the fire department on the radio. They tell us that they are about five miles off the main road and can't move the patient. They also tell us that they haven't been able to find a spot large enough to land the helicopter. Tom acknowledges and tells them that as soon as we spot them, we will look for a place where we can either set down or at least off-load the crew.

By the time the ground crew tells us that they can hear us approaching, I already have the door open and have turned in my seat, and as I'm looking out and down, trying to spot the fire and EMS personnel, a voice comes over the radio. "You're about one mile out," the fireman tells us. I focus about a mile out in front of us, and soon I can see several people on the ground. "There they are!" I tell Tom as I'm pointing. "Ten o'clock, about a half-mile." Instantly, Tom is slowing and putting the ship into a sharp bank to bleed off some airspeed and put the ground crew onto his side of the helicopter so he can start coming up with a plan. As he banks it over to the right, he is looking down through the lower window in his door. "I got 'em!" he tells us. "Okay, I'll start making some orbits, and we can look for a place to land."

I am not having encouraging thoughts about a suitable landing zone, as the ground crew and patient are right in the bottom of a drainage and the canyon walls are not only steep but also filled with very tall pine and fir trees. "Man, this doesn't look good," Bruce says, and we all have to agree. Pretty soon our orbits have grown to where we are about two miles out from the patient, and I speak up. "This is way too far. And we would have to carry him over the hill." Tom speaks up and tells us that he thinks he may have an idea. Bruce and I look at each other, thinking the same thing, *Oh, man! When Tom has an idea, it usually involves screaming and urine.*

"Okay, what?" I ask.

"I saw a granite rock outcropping back near the patient. I think we may be able to do a one skid, let you out, and get the patient in."

"Okay, where did you see that?" I ask.

"Right off our nose. I'll slow down and check out the winds, you look and see if you think we will have enough clearance with the trees and brush."

"Okay, I think I see what you are looking at."

Soon Tom is almost hovering about 150 feet over what looks like a challenging spot, but I think he is right and we will be able to sneak in there, bump the left skid up to the rock, letting one of us out, and get the patient loaded. "I think we can do this," I finally respond. Bruce breaks in and tells us that he will radio the firefighters and EMS crew of the plan and see if they can get the patient up closer to the rock and have him ready for us.

Soon we are orbiting, and looking down, we see that they are indeed moving the patient, who must be on a backboard, to within about twenty feet of where we will be coming down. They radio up that they are ready, and we go over the plan one more time with one another first, then the ground personnel. Once all of us agree, Tom brings the helicopter around, and at first starts his descent right in the middle of the canyon, then as we get closer to the granite area, starts flying the ship sideways to the left closer and closer to the large granite rock. I'm now calling out distances to the rock and also watching under the tail rotor as well as the distance from the ends of the main rotors to the trees, which seem to be getting really close. "Ten feet, eight feet, come down two, six feet, hold that altitude, four feet, two, one." Then just as soon as the three of us feel the skid bump against the rock, I say, "Touchdown!"

Tom takes a few seconds to feel out the ship and how it is balancing on the one point of contact before he feels comfortable enough to tell me, "Okay, go get him." I release my harness and unplug my helmet before stepping out of the helicopter first onto the skid, then onto the rock. I take a quick look back to see Bruce making his way over to my position, kneeling in the doorway. I give him a thumbs-up, and he does the same back to me. At that point, I turn and start over the rock to where the assorted firefighters and ambulance crew are. I can also see a couple of deputy sheriffs and some orange shirts that I assume are county search-and-rescue personnel. As I reach them, we are only about thirty feet away from the hovering helicopter, and I know that most of the helpers will not be able to hear me. I then yell out the instructions. "We are going to carry him up feetfirst. Slide him onto the gurney in the ship. I will work all the controls. Then you all leave the same direction you came, okay?" Everyone nods in agreement. One firefighter is holding up an IV, which I take from him, clamp it off, and lay it on the patient's chest. I see one other volunteer that is still wearing a ball cap and motion for him to take it off. He quickly removes it from his head and simply tosses it away back toward the trail. At that point, I motion with my hands to lift the patient.

The firefighters and EMS crew, in unison, grab the backboard and lift the patient up to their waist. I then motion for them to move forward, and we start moving up and over some assorted boulders to the larger boulder that the helicopter is still balancing on. As we are now under the main rotor blades, I make a motion for all the helpers to bend over, and they do, as if they are all marionettes tied to the same string. When we reach the helicopter, I motion for the person across from me to lift up on his side of the board, which is the foot end. We lift it up and then set it down on the gurney inside the ship, then motion for the rest of the crew to start sliding the patient in, and as they do, I watch the patient's feet and make sure they don't hit anything. As the last firefighter gives the last shove, the patient is on the flight gurney, and I wave for all of them to leave and try to say thank you, which I'm sure no one could hear. Turning back to the ship and working the controls, I roll the patient the rest of the way into the cabin and lock the gurney down.

LONG NIGHT IN BI-COUNTY

Before I climb in, Bruce yells at me to turn on the oxygen. It is located in the rear compartment of the helicopter, and fortunately for us, it is on this same side. I step back now directly under the screaming turbine engine, open the small door, reach in, crank open the oxygen valves, then shut the door. I step back up to the side, and now standing on the skid, I reach in and plug in my helmet. "All good?" I ask as I climb back into my seat.

"Yeah, we're good. Strap your ass down so we can get out of here!" Tom says.

I take a look up at him and can see the concentration and beads of sweat running down his face. He has been holding this very difficult hover against the rock for about five minutes, and I know he must be exhausted.

I snap my seat harness and, turning to look out the open door, tell him, "Okay, we're clear to pull up and away." I watch as the skid leaves the granite and we start up and to the right, slowly sliding away from the mountainside. As we get far enough away, Tom turns the ship to the right and points the nose down the canyon and seems to just let it fall to pick up airspeed. I slide my door closed and start looking at our patient. Bruce is already attaching him to the different monitors, and I plug in the O_2 tubing to the oxygen regulator.

Tom finally breaks the silence. "Well, that was exciting!"

"No shit," I say. "That was a pretty impressive job of hovering, especially from the view I had of being under it, where the patient was. Good job!"

Bruce and I are trying to assess our patient and the different monitors as Tom is making contact with the hospital and giving a short report with our ETA. Before long, we are making our approach to the helipad when Tom tells us that after unloading, he is going for fuel. We acknowledge, and as we set down, we wave the receiving crew up and pull out our patient. As we start down the ramp, Tom takes off, and before we make it to the ready room and elevator, we can barely hear him. As we pull off our helmets, we start up a conversation with our patient. Now that we can actually have a conversation with him, one of the first questions we ask is, "How long have you been having this chest pain?"

ON THE GO

As he starts in on his story, we listen in total amazement. He tells us that he and his wife had hiked into one of their favorite spots in the Strawberry Canyon area yesterday, and just as they were arriving near their destination, he started experiencing this substernal chest pain. He had had a very mild heart attack once in the past and knew right away what was going on and that he needed to get help. He also knew that hiking out himself was out of the question, as it was a fairly vigorous hike. Knowing this, he and his wife decided that she would hike out and get help. This she did, and when she arrived back at her car, she drove a few miles to the nearest payphone and dialed 911. She then told the operator that she would wait at the trailhead and guide the rescuers back in. So at this point, the 911 operator dispatched the local ambulance, Bi-County out of Marysville, and because this was in Plumas County, she dispatched the Plumas County Search and Rescue (SAR) Team.

The woman then returned to the trailhead and waited for the responders, worrying that nothing had happened to her husband. Within about forty-five minutes, the ambulance arrived, and after a short explanation of what was going on and where her husband, the patient, was, the crew grabbed what equipment they thought they would need and started the long hike into the canyon.

By the time the woman and ambulance crew finally arrived at the patient, it was getting late in the evening, around six o'clock, and they knew two things: there was no way they could carry this gentleman out, and it would be dark in about two hours. Looking at their watches, they knew it took them almost an hour to drive to the trailhead and over an hour just to hike in here. After a quick assessment, the paramedic radioed their dispatch and requested an EMS helicopter to respond and fly the patient out. The dispatch center radioed back in a few minutes and told the crew that the Enloe helicopter was en route and would be there in about thirty minutes. The patient then tells us that the ambulance crew was taking care of him and explaining that one of them also works part-time at Enloe and is very familiar with their helicopter and crew, then tells him, "If anyone can get you out of here, it will be them."

At that point, the patient felt very relaxed and was trying to calm his wife. The paramedics and EMT were watching their cardiac monitor and making sure they would have enough oxygen to last until the helicopter arrived. When they decided the helicopter should now only be about ten minutes out, the crew was starting to package him up a little when several people came out of the brush from the trail. They were all a little stunned to see these people and soon realized they were personnel from the Plumas County Search and Rescue.

The paramedic rose to great them and, knowing the helicopter was about ten minutes out, started filling them in on what his plan was. Before he could finish, the sheriff deputy in charge of search and rescue cut him off, telling him, "No, we aren't going to do that." He then keyed up his radio and told his dispatch to cancel the Enloe helicopter, and he wanted to put in a request for the rescue helicopter from the US Navy stationed at Fallon Naval Air Station in Nevada to do a long-line extraction.

The paramedic and sheriff deputy almost immediately got into a verbal disagreement, the paramedic stating that he already had a plan, the helicopter was almost here, and he was in charge of the patient. The deputy then argued that he was in charge of all SAR missions and it was up to him how this patient would be taken out. According to our patient, this argument went on for some time and not only became quite vocal but also almost physical a couple of times and would only end when the deputy threatened to put the paramedic in handcuffs if he wouldn't shut up.

Bruce and I can't believe the story we are hearing. We also know that this explains why we were canceled yesterday, and we tell our patient that we were the ones working yesterday as well and knew about the cancellation. By now the two of us are very intrigued with the story and want to hear the rest of it, but we have arrived in the ED and the cardiologist wants to examine him and do whatever he needs to. We tell him that we will let him go for now but will follow up after he gets admitted to the floor. Bruce and I leave him in good hands, and as we gather equipment to restock the helicopter and do our report, we discuss the possible ordeals that we think our patient must have gone through, but still don't understand why it took them twenty-four hours to call us back.

A few hours later, one of the receptionists calls us out to the front desk. We arrive to find our patient's wife, who has finally made it to the hospital after her three-mile hike out and long drive to Chico. Bruce and I decide to escort her up to the cardiac care unit (CCU) and maybe hear the rest of the story. As we are riding up in the elevator, we fill in the wife on what her husband has told us, and just as we are getting to the part about the verbal argument between the sheriff deputy and the paramedic, we enter into his room. The wife is really glad to see him and wants to know what all they've done. Of course, Bruce and I want to skip all that and get back to the story, but a little compassion kicks in and we let him tell her that he was taken to the cath lab, and when she asks questions about that procedure, we help answer what they do there.

Finally, not able to hold back any further, and just as we are pulling up a chair for the wife and a couple of chairs for us, Bruce asks, "Okay, so did the paramedic and sheriff get into it?"

Laughing, both the wife and husband say, "Almost." He then starts up the story again where he left off.

It took almost two hours for the sheriff department to get base approval from the commander of the naval air station to send the helicopter to a civilian rescue, but they did. When the helicopter arrived, there were about thirty minutes of daylight left. When the ship appeared overhead, neither the wife nor the husband could believe what they were looking at. It was one of the biggest helicopters in the Navy inventory, a CH-47 Chinook. Twin rotors, loud enough to be heard from about one hundred miles away. The wife then adds that when the helicopter started orbiting over them, the amount of downwash from the large rotors was throwing an enormous amount of debris, bushes, and branches from trees onto all the workers below.

As the large helicopter started its hover, a door opened from under the belly of the ship, and soon, squinting to keep debris out of their eyes, they could see someone with a helmet on looking down at them through this door. At the same time, they were radioing instructions to the SAR personnel that they would lower the basket to them attached to a winch inside the helicopter that deployed down through this door. When they got the basket, they were to place the patient in it, lying supine on his back. They would then raise the basket with the winch until he was safely inside. The SAR people were trying to now tell our patient how this was going to happen, and he tells us that he was not excited about this in the least bit. Being hoisted up in the air was not what he had planned on, and at the same time, the argument with the paramedic and deputy started up again. The paramedic was now yelling that all this was not needed and, in fact, might worsen any heart attack he might be having from all the anxiety he was going to have during the hoist. The deputy just ignored him.

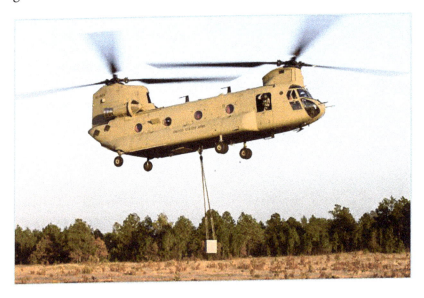

Within a few minutes, they could see the basket being lowered, and after it was on the ground, the SAR personnel were moving him over and securing him into it. He remembers one of them telling him, "We do this all the time." He really didn't feel reassured, and before he could let anyone know that he had changed his mind, the line tightened and he started up.

The wife then takes over the story, telling us that as she and all the fire, EMS, SAR, and deputy watched as he was being lifted the approximately 150 feet to the helicopter, it suddenly stopped about halfway.

The wife tells us that she watched in horror as the helicopter was just hovering, the basket no longer being winched up, and now it had started spinning. Soon it was spinning faster and faster. She became ill, thinking of what her husband was going through, and finally started yelling at the deputy to do something. The deputy was finally contacted by the pilot to tell them that the winch had broken. They couldn't pull it up and were going to see if it would go down. If so, they would lower the patient back down to them. At that point, they did start lowering the basket, and all the people on the ground were hoping that nothing worse would happen, that the entire package wouldn't just let go and he would fall.

After what seemed to be an eternity, the basket made it back down to the rescuers and they were able to grab it and stop its death spin, placing it on the ground and detaching it from the line. After the pilot was informed he was free, the helicopter then lifted, with the cable hanging loose below it. The pilot told them they would fly to the nearest base, which was Beal AFB in Marysville, and see if they could fix it.

As the helicopter finally left the scene and was far enough out of hearing range so the people on the ground could talk once again, everyone looked around at one another to see if anyone had any ideas. At this time, it was also noticed that everyone was covered in dirt and dust and had muddy lines on their faces where tears from their eyes had been trying to flush out dirt and was just running down their dirt-covered faces. Then, once again, the deputy and paramedic started yelling at each other on what was going to happen next. The problem was, it was now dark. They knew there was no way a helicopter was going to fly into the canyon until sunup, and everyone knew that they were going to have to spend the night.

Someone started a fire as the paramedic and EMT stayed with the patient, checking vital signs every thirty minutes and only turning on the cardiac monitor once each hour to look at his rhythm.

The EMT finally gave up on the oxygen after about three hours, as he had been turning it down, then it finally ran out. At that point, he removed the nasal cannula and just tossed the entire works aside.

The wife then tells us that when they originally walked into the canyon, they really didn't plan on spending the night, and even with the fire going, they were dressed in shorts and T-shits and froze their butts off.

At this point, I am adding up the time they had been there, and knowing we didn't pick them up until the following evening, I ask, "So when the sun came up, what took so long for them to call us back?"

The couple looked at each other, shaking their heads, then the wife tells us that at daybreak, the deputy told everyone that the Navy was still trying to fix the winch or replace it. They also said, if they couldn't get it fixed in a few hours, they would send a different helicopter.

"Where was that one going to come from?" I ask.

"Well, that was one of the other problems. They weren't sure where another one with a winch was located, maybe the Coast Guard from San Francisco." The both of them then tell us that as we could imagine, the arguments went on all day long between the paramedic and the sheriff deputy, almost becoming physical several times. The Navy would call the sheriff dispatcher, she would pass along updates, and the fight would be back on. There always seemed to be another delay.

Finally, around six o'clock the second evening, the paramedic radioed his dispatch and requested the Enloe helicopter once again. This time, he told his dispatcher to relay to the Enloe dispatcher that for no reason except from a call from him personally will the helicopter be canceled, especially from the sheriff's office. The couple grin then tell us that at that point, the deputy started yelling at the paramedic and the paramedic finally told him that if he wanted to stop him, he would have to pull his gun out and shoot him. That there was no way he was going to spend another night in the canyon just to fulfill his ego. Laughing, the couple then tell us that for a moment, the deputy had his hand on his gun and they actually thought he was going to pull it out. At that point, the paramedic and deputy were standing face-to-face, eye to eye, in a final showdown. The deputy finally turned away and back to his personnel, saying that the paramedic had no idea what he was doing. The deputy then got back onto his radio and was trying to get an ETA on the Navy helicopter, hoping it would be in the air soon, but he was told it would be several more hours.

About thirty minutes later, they heard our helicopter overhead and said they couldn't believe it when it dropped down into the canyon and hovered with the one skid on the rock and I got out. Then when I knelt down to talk to the patient, they said they knew they were in good hands and just might get out of there. The wife then tells us, as she watched us carry her husband up the rock and put him in the helicopter, she was amazed, and when we lifted away and she saw me for the last time waving to the crew below, she knew her husband was finally in good hands, and broke down and cried.

I turn to look at Bruce, and at the same time, he is looking back at me, and both of our jaws are open. We simply can't believe the story we've just heard. I turn my head a little further and look at the door to our room behind us and notice that there is a crowd of nursing staff that has gathered and has also been listening to the story, including my Drena. I stand up and, looking at the crowd, say, "Don't you have something else you should be doing?" They all laugh and then, amazingly, all start to clap.

One of them then speaks up, saying, "That was the best story I've heard in a long time."

As the staff start to leave and go back to their own patients, I drag my chair out of the room and stop when I get to the last remaining staff, Drena. She only stands in my way, looking at me eye to eye, smiling. Then she says, "My hero!"

"Let's get out of here," I say to her as we turn, and I put the chair back at the nursing station.

She accompanies me out of the CCU and to the elevator. As we ride it down to the first floor, we talk about how amazing it is that some people have horrible ordeals and their story never gets told. I also tell her I wonder if the ambulance crew and sheriff department will critique this call as a lesson learned. What to do and what not to do in similar cases. Of course, neither one of us will ever know that answer.

She has her arm looped through one of mine as we walk through the door to the emergency department. I ask her what time she thinks she will be taking a lunch break, and before she can answer, my pager starts beeping. "FlightCare, scene flight, I-5. Heading two eight zero, forty miles."

We stop.

She squeezes a little harder, telling me, "Be careful. I want that lunch date."

"You got it!" I answer, then let go, our arms slowly sliding apart, and when our hands meet, we pause, giving each other one last squeeze before I turn back to the elevator.

6

WRONG WAY, TONY

IT'S SO FOGGY out that I almost get lost trying to drive to work. As I'm trying to find clues along the back streets of Chico that look familiar to me and make the correct turns, I can see how disorienting it can be. At the same time, I am thinking that I hope they put us flight crew on an ambulance tonight so we can at least have a possibility of escape from the ED. Maybe a motor vehicle accident in downtown Chico or a long transfer to Sacramento. Although a transfer to Sacramento in this fog could be a twelve-hour ride. Okay, maybe not Sacramento.

    I finally arrive in the parking lot at Enloe, find a space, and make my way toward the glow that I know must be the ambulance entrance. As I start up the walkway, I can make out a couple of ambulances parked on the ramp and know it is going to be a busy night. As the sliding glass doors start to open, I can hear the unmistakable sounds of the ED, nurses running around; the charge nurse trying to catch them as they pass, wanting to know when more beds will be opening up, the nurses just holding their hands up as if to say, "Hell if I know"; patients moaning, some crying, others leaning on the counter at the nurse's station, wanting answers as to when their significant other will be seen. Another is saying that if he could just get a new Dilaudid prescription to replace the one he lost, he could leave, and all of them want to know, "What the hell is taking so long?" Of course, the nursing staff is too busy to answer, and the secretary has no idea and only tells them to return to their room and the nurse will be there shortly.

Ugh, I think to myself. I am now really hoping we can be put on an ambulance. I instantly start to think of a good reason to tell the charge nurse why we should be on an ambulance. *I think my best bet is that because of the fog, there may be too many calls at once for the first-out rigs to handle and we will be needed,* AND *if there is an interfacility, we will already have checked out our assigned rig and will be ready to go.* Yes, that's it! I will now just have to make it sound believable. As I walk through the hallway, making my way to the lounge to meet up with the day crew, I pass through what we commonly refer to as the gurney garage. It's an overflow of patients. Once the beds fill up in the regular areas of the ED, the spare gurneys that line the hallway will start filling up with the overflow. It can be very challenging maneuvering through these, as some of the patients are wanting to talk to anyone that passes; some are tied down to the gurney, while some are handcuffed. You also must be careful where you step, as some beds have urine running off one end, some have vomit, and some have both. I can see the mop bucket standing at the ready and know that it has already been used a few times, as the liquid in the bucket no longer looks or smells of a cleaning detergent but something you may smell from under the bridge in town or the alley behind one of the bars.

As I enter the lounge and spot my fellow crew members, I can't help but announce myself and my analysis of the sights and sounds I've just walked through. "Please tell me we can be on an ambulance!" I stand in the door as the crew turns their heads and grins, knowing exactly what I want. One of them speaks up and, in a slightly laughing voice, says, "No way! We tried. They said we had to stay because it was too busy." Dang, this is not what I want to hear. I stand with the look of desperation on my face as the door slowly closes behind me, then ask what they've tried so I can attempt something else. The day crew then tells me several reasons they tried, all of which included a good amount of whining, but all were unsuccessful. Just as I am concentrating on what techniques I should try, our night charge nurse walks into the lounge. I hold the door open for him, and before he can get all his evening greetings out, I start in on him. With my best we-need-to-do-this-or-people-will-die expressions, I ask him, "Hey, can we be on the backup ambulance tonight? It looks really busy and the first-out crew may be overwhelmed, and there is a good possibility of a critical care transfer tonight, and if we are already assigned and have the rig checked, we could get out of here faster. What do you think?"

There is dead silence in the room; the day shift is slightly impressed with my ability to sound professional and whine all in the same sentence. The charge nurse has paused in his routine and is staring at me, not saying anything. This I take as a good sign—at least he is thinking about it. It usually doesn't take long to say no. Finally, resuming his routine of putting his lunch in the refrigerator, setting his bag down, and heading toward the lounge door, which I am now standing in front of, he stops and, knowing I want an answer before I step out of the way, looks at me, takes a breath, and says, "Sure, why not?"

I step out of the way so he can leave and get his report from the day charge nurse, and just before the door fully closes, I make a fist with my hand and, pulling it from the air down to my waist, let out an enthusiastic, "Yeeeesss!"

Immediately the day shift starts in on me. "I can't believe you talked him into that!" Obviously, they are a little perturbed that we may have a chance to get out of here when they didn't. "We should go talk to him and tell him that you should stay and spend the entire evening mopping the urine and puke in the gurney garage."

"NO WAY!" I respond with a big grin on my face as I set my bags down. Then to add a little salt into their wounds, I add, "Excuse us, but we have to go preflight our ambulance!" As my partner, Neal, and I make our way through the door, leaving the day crew, we know they are too polite to give us the bird but also know they are thinking it.

We check in with the charge paramedic to let him know we will be available, and he is glad to hear it. He assigns us a rig and a driver, and the three of us make our way out through the fog to check the ambulance. We know the chances of us having a run are slim, as the other crews will respond if they are not already committed, and we also know the greatest chance of a run is if a neighboring hospital has a patient that they need transferred and would normally call the helicopter.

    We have finished with the checks and have been given some assignments back in the ED to help out the nursing staff. It is a fairly busy night, and before I know it, it is past two in the morning. I am finally able to get a break and decide to go to the cafeteria to sit and relax. I make my way downstairs and shuffle through the salad bar. I see some friends from another part of the hospital at a table and decide to sit and talk with them. As I take a seat, they are already asking if the ED is busy. They want to know if they may be getting any more admits. I decide to mess with them and tell them, "I think you may. There is a guy upstairs that has uncontrolled vomiting and diarrhea for the last week and should be admitted as soon as they find a doctor to accept him." They look at me with a questioning look on their faces, as if they are not certain if I am serious or pulling their legs. I see this and decide to add to this patient's story. "No, really! As soon as they get the toxicology report back and have a diagnosis of either unknown autoimmune disorder, acute syphilis, gonorrheamegaly, or just penile discharge of unknown etiology, they will send him to you."

    I have been able to tell them all this without breaking into a smile. Two of the nurses have decided to just ignore me, knowing I'm messing with them; the other two are fish on the line. Soon, they have taken the bait and are asking more about their mystery patient. "What do you think it is?" one of the female nurses asks.

    "I don't really know," I answer, then add, "I understand that there is some strange sexually transmitted disease being passed around Chico State in the dorms. This is probably one of them." At this point, one of the older nurses knows I'm bullshitting them and also knows I'm baiting the younger nurse on, and he is smiling as he eats his meal, shaking his head. As the young nurse asks more questions, all in a row, not giving me a chance to answer any of them, my pager starts beeping.

    As I stand up from the table, I shovel a couple more forkfuls of salad into my mouth, and as I'm turning to leave, the young nurse is still asking questions. At this point, all I can do with a mouthful of chef salad is to attempt to let out some mumbled words that I know are not understandable. I dump the remainder of the salad into the trash can and quickly set my tray onto the dumbwaiter. A quick look back at the table, and I can see the young nurse with a puzzled look on her face and the others smiling, knowing I've pulled one off on her.

I start jogging down the hallway and bypass the elevators, knowing I can just run up the stairway at the west entrance and that will put me right outside the ED. As I open the door, Neal and our driver, Tony, have already made it to the rig and are climbing in.

"What's up?" I ask as I climb into the back, looking into the front at the two of them.

"Chest pain patient," Neal tells me as he is writing down our time out.

Tony then adds, "Somewhere south of town." He then asks Neal if he will help look up the address on one of the maps, as not only is he unfamiliar with the address, but he also can't see anything that is not twenty feet in front of him in the dense fog. Neal tells him to just head south out of town and he will contact the fire department to get some better directions.

Tony is leaning forward against the steering wheel, as if being four inches from the windshield is going to make him see better. Soon, Neal has the fire engine company on the radio, and they are giving us some directions as to where they are. From my rear seat, I can see nothing. It all looks like a sea of white haze with red lights flashing back into our faces. I have been able to tell that we have left the city, and after what has only been about fifteen minutes but seems to be an hour, we have made several turns and somehow arrive at a residence with a big red fire engine sitting outside. Neal has done the impossible, and before we exit the rig, I give him an attaboy by telling him, "Nice instrument flying!" He just smiles and meets me at the back door to help carry in some of the equipment.

We enter the home knowing we have already determined I will be the primary caregiver and Neal will be gathering the family information from the relatives. As I work my way to the back bedroom, where the patient is, the first thing I see is that it is really dark. I see a couple of firefighters standing by the bed, and they appear to be talking to someone sitting up on the bed. As I make my way to the front of the patient, I ask one of the firefighters if they could find some more light. At that point, the other firefighter gives me a report of what he knows. As he is telling me the patient's age, medical history, and vital signs, I am attaching the cardiac monitor. I can see he is already on oxygen, but in the dark room, something just doesn't look right. As I'm listening to the firefighter's report, which seems to be really long, for some reason, and at the same time squinting to look at the patient's face, I've placed my hand on the patient's wrist to feel for a pulse, and although there is one, it feels really weak. At the same time, Neal, who has been in the other room, talking to family, sticks his head in the room, asking if I need anything. I tell him I am just starting but need more light. He then turns around to talk to the wife again, as she has returned to him with what seems to be an Easter basket full of the patient's medications.

I decide to quit listening to the firefighter's verbal report, as I have a bad feeling about my patient, and even as the firefighter continues to talk, I start asking the patient how he is doing. He is just staring at me with a gaze that seems to be looking right through me at death itself. I take a quick glance at the monitor, and it has a very fast sinus tachycardic rhythm. I am not getting much out of the patient, and after a quick assessment of lung sounds and a finding of edema in the patient's legs, I decide to hurry with getting an IV established and let Neal know that we need to get the hell out of here.

I push the angiocath under the patient's skin and see the blood flash in the end of the catheter. At the same time, I can hear Neal giving a patient report to the base hospital. He is unable to pronounce some of the medications' names and is now spelling them out. As I am attaching the IV line to the catheter, I can now feel the patient starting to pull away from me. I tell him to not move as I'm reaching for the small pieces of tape that I had already torn and placed on my thigh. He continues to slowly pull his arm, and I am now concentrating on not losing my IV and verbalize a little louder, "Don't move, please!" I then look up from my IV site to give a little facial expression to add to this point when, in the darkness of the room, I notice the patient slowly slumping to the side, his eyes now glossed over.

I grab his shoulder, and a quick look at the cardiac monitor shows me exactly what I've feared: he is now in V-fib. He has coded on me. "Shit!" I yell out to the remaining firefighters, then add, "Quick, lay him down and start CPR!" As I am reaching for the defibrillation pads on the monitor and attaching them to the patient's chest, the firefighters are pulling the patient off the bed onto the floor and have started chest compressions. Just then, Neal has taken a break from his spelling bee, and as he pops his head back into the room, asking, "How's it going?" I answer with a "CLEAR!"

The energy hits the patient's chest, and he tightens up and bounces about six inches off the floor. Neal is now entering the room and asks, "What the hell happened?"

"He just coded," I tell him, then add, "He was never verbal. He sounded like crap. I believe he is in heart failure."

I shock the patient another time, and his rhythm changes back to a sinus tach, but there is a lot of PVCs (premature ventricular contractions), and I know this won't last long without some intervention. Neal has made his way to the patient's head and is setting up to intubate him, and I'm pulling the lidocaine out of the bag, popping off the yellow caps, screwing the vial to the needle, and pushing the medication into the IV line. Just as Neal is telling me he has the tube in, I see that the patient has gone back into V-fib. I tell the firefighters to start CPR again as I charge up the defibrillator. As it is charging, I tell the fire captain, who has joined us in the room, to get a backboard and help us get him out of here.

"CLEAR!" I yell, and the firefighters and Neal both step back from the patient's side just before I push the button. The patient once again bounces off the floor, and looking back at the monitor, I see he has once again gone back to a sinus tach. As one of the firefighters takes over the airway, Neal, Tony, and I grab all our equipment, and the other two firefighters grab the patient and, in one big movement, pull him off the floor onto the backboard and not stopping until we set it down on the gurney in the hallway. We then start out through the living room, down the walkway, and into the back of the ambulance. Just as we latch the gurney to the floor, I see he has gone into V-fib again. As I reach for the monitor to charge up the pads, I ask the fire captain if one of the firefighters can ride with us as we may need him. He agrees and tells one of the firefighters that is an EMT to get in with us. As he climbs in, I have finished my defibrillation and see that it doesn't have any effect. I tell the firefighter to start CPR, and as Tony is closing the doors, asking if we need anything, all I say is, "Let's get out of here."

As the ambulance is now bouncing down the road, Neal and I are beyond busy. We are pushing a host of different medications, trying to stabilize the patient's heart rhythm. The firefighter is trying his best to continue with CPR compressions as he is being tossed around with each bump in the road, right turn, left turn, and sudden application of the brakes as Tony is seeing all kinds of spooky things trying to jump out in front of him as he makes his way through the incredibly thick fog.

Soon, Neal and I are getting a little concerned. We have given just about every medication that we have in the rig and have even pulled out the backup medication box to keep up with our demands, and the hospital is calling and asking for an update. I tell them that CPR is still in progress, everything we have done, and as I turn in the seat, looking forward into the cab and out the windshield, trying to make out some landmark to give them an ETA, I see a sign appearing out of the fog. Squinting, staring, trying to make out what it says, and when it finally comes out of the fog and into the headlights, I read, DURHAM CITY LIMIT.

"TONY!" I yell. "Turn around! You're going the wrong way!" I can't believe it. Somewhere after leaving the patient's house, he made a left turn instead of a right turn and, being totally disoriented in the dense fog, had been heading south when he should have been heading north. Finally, mustering up enough courage to speak, he asks, "Are you sure?"

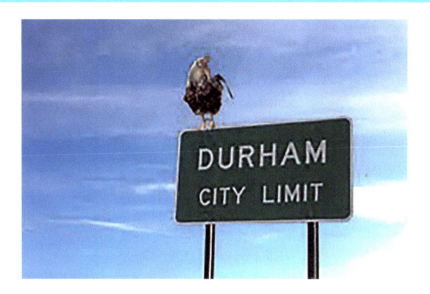

"What do you mean am I sure?" It is now obvious as we pull up to a stop sign right in front of the Durham store. "We just pulled into Durham! Turn around and get us to Chico!" I insist.

As I turn back to the patient, Neal asks what is going on, and I inform him that we've just entered Durham. He replies with a "You've got to be kidding me?"

"Nope," I answer, and within a few seconds, we can all feel Tony bringing the ambulance to a stop and flipping a U-turn. "Unbelievable" is all I can say as I sit in the jump seat, holding the microphone, thinking how I'm going to update the hospital that our ETA has changed from what I thought was five minutes to now around twenty-five to thirty minutes.

I key up the radio and relay the new information about our ETA. Immediately, the hospital wants to know why the new, extended ETA, and I decide I don't want to broadcast the error over the radio into scanner land for everyone in the county to hear. A simple "I'll explain when we get there" will have to work.

I hang the radio back up and ask Neal where he would like me to help. During the ride back to Chico, Neal, the firefighter, and I have all switched off with the duty of chest compressions and ventilating the patient. By the time we hit the city limits, we are completely out of drugs. Neal asks me what we have left that we could give, and looking into the drug box and after shuffling through a few items, I answer back, "Well, if you think he may be having a miscarriage, we could give him some Pitocin, but otherwise, I think we're done." We both chuckle a little, and I try to look out one of the windows to figure out where we are. All I can see is the glow of lights through the fog and really don't have a clue of our location. I finally ask Tony, "Any idea where we are and when we'll be at Enloe?"

"Well," he answers, "I think we should be there in about five minutes." Straining through the windshield, he then continues, "The problem is, it is really hard to see the street names, and I am just hoping that I don't miss a turn." I don't want to be sarcastic and add salt into his wounds with a comment like, "You mean like the last turn you missed," but decide he already feels bad about the incident.

I turn my attention back to Neal and the patient. As they look at me for an answer, I just shake my head and hold up my hands as if to say, "No idea!" Within a few more minutes, I can tell we have turned off the road and are climbing up the ambulance ramp. As Tony puts the rig into park, the rear doors open and we are greeted by two of the nurses and the ED doctor.

"Where the hell have you been?" simultaneously comes out their mouths.

"We missed a turn," I answer and then try to get everyone to focus on the patient and just get him out of the rig and into the ED so we can decide what to do next.

As we transfer him off the ambulance gurney and onto the emergency department gurney, the ED physician places his fingers at first on the patient's neck, searching for a pulse and asking us how long it has been since we have had a rhythm. "Been some time," we answer as we look at our watches, trying to figure out an exact answer to his question. The physician then puts his stethoscope on and, listening to the patient's chest, attempts to auscultate any heart tones. Neal and I finally decide that it has been about forty-five minutes minimum since we have had any pulse or rhythm. The doctor takes a step back and, knowing that we have given him every drug in our inventory without success, takes one last look at the monitor and says, "That's it, he's gone." Turning to the nurse that is recording on the emergency department form, he then asks, "What time do you have?" The nurse then tells him the time, and they agree on the time of death.

Neal and I then get together and try to come up with what we are going to do about the call. We know we have to restock and write the patient care report but then try to decide if we need to write up a hospital incident report. Still undecided, we ask the charge nurse, and he agrees that we should. None of us like writing these, and we know it will launch an investigation, and eventually someone's butt will be on the line. We know Tony already feels bad enough about it, but I decide to tell him that I have to write it up and he will more than likely be getting a visit from the boss in a few days. He totally understands and tells both of us that he is really sorry about the incident. We tell him not to worry about it too much but in the future, if he is unsure about where we are or where to go, to ask someone. A quick slap on the shoulder, and we go about our business of restocking the rig and writing the report.

I arrive to work a week later to find the ambulance coordinator waiting for me. I smile in passing, and as I walk down the hall to the lockers, he joins me. I know he is here to interview me about the call, and after we talk for a while, I finally tell him that looking from the outside, it does look really bad, but in Tony's defense, it was foggier than shit that night. He then tells me that he agrees it was an unfortunate incident and he has already spoken with Tony and knows he feels really bad. He then asks if I think the patient's outcome would have been any different if we had gotten here earlier. I take a moment to think about my answer and, shaking my head, say, "No, there really isn't anything that I believe would have been done here in the ED that we didn't do in the ambulance." Then I add, "And by the time we ran out of medications to give, I'm pretty certain that the ED doc would have pronounced the patient anyway. There really wasn't anything more anyone could have done." He thinks about it for a moment, then agrees and tells me he will finish his report and eventually get me a copy. We shake hands and go our separate ways. I run into Neal later and ask if he has been interviewed, and he tells me he has. We then wonder if anything like this has happened in the past, and when asking any of the other ambulance crews, the answer seems to be the same. "No!"

Somehow I don't believe all of them.

7

CHESTER SNOWMOBILE

"**CAN YOU GET** into trouble for doing your job?" I am asked this question by students all the time. My answer usually explains that with every scenario they will see in their career, more than likely, it cannot be found in a book; sometimes you have to make the best choice on the information you have at the time, and if your intention is to help someone, you should be covered legally. Although, sometimes you are faced with a real dilemma of "Which choice will get me into the least amount of trouble?" A sample of this would be if you arrive at the scene of a vehicular accident and you are directed to a patient that is covered in blood and is telling you and everyone, "I'm fine, leave me alone." A person has the right to refuse treatment, so unless you can prove that they are not of sound mind, maybe intoxicated or a head injury, and not making a sound decision, you will have to decide to leave them alone as they are requesting or strap them down to a board and transport them for treatment. If you leave them alone and they die in the taxi on the way home, you will definitely be in trouble; if you take them to the hospital and they only have a small laceration on their scalp and say they will sue you for taking them against their will, can you be sued? You can't be sued for doing the right thing or, more importantly, the intent of doing the right thing. If it gets to court, the judge or jury will side with the difficult decisions we have to make and, without diagnostic equipment on scene to rule out a head injury, will probably cite the rule of implied consent, which is, "What would the prudent patient want if they were making sound decisions?" And the answer would be to be treated and transported.

Some of my biggest issues in this category always happen when someone's ego is involved. You already read about "Long Night in Bi-County." The ego was the deputy sheriff who wanted to do things his way; he was a big intimidating guy and had a gun. It took twenty-four hours before the medic told him to just get the hell out of the way or pull his gun and shoot him. The deputy really had no reason for trying to take control of the scene and overriding the paramedic, as he wasn't in charge of the patient, but he wanted to do things his way but should have worked with the paramedic instead to unite on one plan and make it happen. I usually try very hard to work with people like this, and fortunately, this doesn't happen very often. Usually, the two of you can discuss the problem and come up with a scenario that will work best for the both of you.

Fast-forward about three years. I'm still working on the helicopter, and the same deputy is still the same deputy with an ego problem.

I arrive at work in the evening, wondering what I'll be doing tonight. It is January, and we know that there is a lot of snow in the mountains. The mechanic has put the snow skids on the helicopter, and it is always fun to fly up to the mountains and land in the snow.

Shortly after we finish our preflight, we ride the elevator back down to the ED and check in with the charge nurse. She gives us some assignments, and we get to work helping out where we can. So far this evening, I have had some really interesting patients and probably have spent too much time chatting with them about what they do or answering questions about the helicopter. I always like to ask the college students what their major is, what they are studying, and if they like it. I have asked one patient what he wants to do, and I can tell he is really not focused. He tells me he is just taking his general education classes right now and knows he needs to declare a major soon, when his girlfriend suddenly interrupts him and speaks up. "I want to be a nurse!"

"Really? Well, what do you want to know about nursing?" I ask, as I like to talk to someone that has a goal, is focused, and knows what she really wants. As she starts telling me that she wants to finish school, start working here at Enloe, and eventually end up in the emergency department, and possibly on the helicopter, I can't help but wonder why she is with this guy, who really has no goal in life.

I start to fill her in that nursing is really a good job, not just in taking care of people but that there is an endless career ladder and a job in every town. I can see her lighting up to the idea as I sell the position and give her some pointers on how to further her career once she graduates from nursing school. Now wide-eyed, she asks me what it is like to be a flight nurse. I think for a moment, glancing at her looser boyfriend, then turn back to her and state, "It is the most exciting thing you can do with your pants on!" The girl is blushing and chuckling, now hooked on the career, as she knows that is what she wants to do, and the boyfriend has a smirk on his face. And then, as if right on cue, my pager starts beeping. I can see that the young nursing student is now overwhelmed with excitement as I start taking my gloves off as the audible comes over the radio. "FlightCare, scene flight. Snowmobile accident north of Chester, heading zero one zero degrees at fifty-five miles." I quickly finish up what I'm doing and have the boyfriend sign his discharge instructions, give him his copy, and set the remainder of the chart down to finish when I get back. As I start walking away, I can tell the girl wants to chase me down, wanting to know more about what the call is, where we are going, what will we do when we get there, and many more question. I just smile as I'm walking away and tell her, "Just keep studying. You'll get there."

I reach the elevator and meet up with Mike and Tom. We all step in, and as we are riding up, we start talking about where we may be going. I take my horse up to this area often during the summer to camp out and ride in the Caribou Wilderness. It is just northeast of Chester and borders the east side of Lassen Volcanic National Park. A beautiful area to simply get lost in. I am sure there are a lot of snowmobilers that ride in this area in the winter, as I see the parking lot full on the weekends when I'm up there, working at the fire department.

As we are buckling into the helicopter, I ask dispatch if they can give us a better location. They get back to us that the ambulance is requesting us and currently they are in the parking lot at the south entrance to the wilderness. I tell Tom that I know this area and exactly where they are.

As we lift from the rooftop, I still have my sliding door open and take a look down at the parking lot in front of the emergency entrance. To my surprise, I see the nursing student and her boyfriend walking out of the hospital, and she is looking up and waving at us. I smile and send a big wave back to her before sliding the door closed.

As we are making our way toward Chester, dispatch gets back to us that the county search-and-rescue team is also en route. We acknowledge this, knowing that the ambulance wouldn't have snowmobiles and there is a chance we may be setting down in the parking lot with the ambulance until the search-and-rescue unit finds the patient and, more than likely, brings the patient out to us.

As we crest the ridge and start across Chester then Lake Almanor, I radio the ambulance and update them that we are about five minutes out from their location. They acknowledge us and tell us that they are indeed sitting in the parking lot, which I've expected, and inform us that search-and-rescue is responding from Quincy and is not here yet. They then ask if we can fly the road into the wilderness and look for the patient. We agree to this after they tell us that one of the parties that is with this group states the patient is about five miles in on the main road. Just as he is finishing telling us this, I look down and can see the ambulance in the parking lot and point it out to Tom. Tom also sees them and the main road leading up the hill. It really sticks out, as all the trees are dark green and the road is solid white, like someone has drawn a white line on a black chalkboard.

We start up the road and, within a few minutes, come across several snowmobiles and people all waving frantically at us. Tom starts an orbit around the scene. As I slide the door open to get a better look, I can see someone lying on the ground, covered with coats and blankets.

"Yup, this must be it," I say over the intercom, and I can also tell that Tom is slowing and starting to make an approach into the scene. "You going to put it on the road?" I ask.

"Yup, just short of the snowmobilers. I'm pretty sure the road is going to be packed from all the riders. Just make sure we don't start sliding off the road once we put down."

"Copy that," I reply, then start calling out our distances to the ground.

Landing in snow can be a little tricky for the first-time pilot, but Tom and I have done it many times and know what we have to do without telling each other. We will slowly get close enough to the ground that the rotor wash will start stirring up the snow. Trouble is, if you try to set down into this, you will be in what is commonly referred to as a whiteout. You will not be able to see past the windshield and then will lose your orientation and can land on your side or fly into a tree. The best thing to do is hover at a safe distance that you can leave if you have to and let the rotor wash blow all the loose snow up and away until it is clear enough that you can see the ground once again.

Once we accomplish this, I let Tom know I can see the ground and he can continue to set down. He slowly lowers the helicopter until the skis come into contact with the road. We sit there for a moment, feeling out the helicopter, making sure there isn't enough slope for it to start sliding. When we are finally comfortable, Tom idles the engine down and Mike and I step out, carrying our gear toward the group of people.

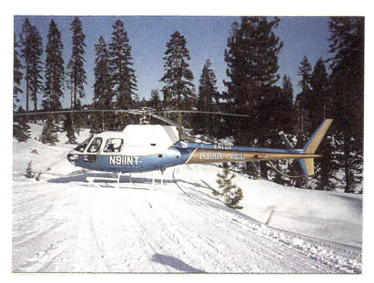

CHESTER SNOWMOBILE

As we walk up to the group, one of the men walks up to us, saying, "Man, are we glad to see you!"

"What happened?" I ask him as I start surveying the scene. The man starts talking as we are walking up to a woman lying on the ground. Pointing to a large green pipe gate that the Forest Service uses to close off roads in the winter, he tells us that all of them were moving along at a pretty good speed of around 45 to 50 miles per hour when they came around the corner and suddenly saw the gate that was buried below the snow but, because of some warm days and the snow melting, is now about one foot above the packed surface. He continues to tell me that most of the riders were able to make quick adjustments and miss the gate, but the woman got a ski caught up in a track and couldn't turn, then they all watched as she hit it at full speed.

Looking at the gate, I can see that it has a pretty good bend in it, and given the fact that it is about a four-inch piece of pipe, this is pretty impressive. I can now also see the snowmobile that hit the gate; there are pieces scattered everywhere, and it is most certainly destroyed.

Now turning my attention to the woman on the ground, Mike and I start assessing her. She is about thirty years old. She does tell me that she remembers what happened, and I can tell she is in an incredible amount of pain and seems short of breath. Mike is checking her out below the waist as I listen to her lungs. After the two of us finish with our own assessments, we tell each other what we have found as the two of us start putting her on oxygen and starting an IV. Between the two of us, we have found that she has multiple fractured ribs and probably a collapsed lung. Mike tells me that she also has a fractured pelvis and left femur. Tom has joined us, and we tell him we need to C-spine the woman. We decide to not put her leg into a traction device because of the pelvic fracture, but instead, we put the KED upside down around her pelvis, with the neck portion around her fractured leg. This actually works out really well, and we are able to then move her onto our gurney and, with the help of the other snowmobilers, carry her and load her into the helicopter.

We thank the snowmobile party for helping us then ask them to step away as Tom starts up the ship. With a quick wave, I slide the door closed before Tom pulls power so we aren't covered with snow. After Tom lifts off, he radios the ambulance crew still waiting in the snow park that we indeed have the patient and are en route back to Enloe.

The trip back to Chico is fairly busy. We are trying to start a second IV and keep an eye on her respirations, knowing she may develop a tension pneumothorax at any time, but we also know that decreasing in altitude will help her, and in fact it does. By the time we get over Chico, she is breathing much better but is still in a lot of pain from all the fractures.

Tom drops us off on the heliport, as usual, then heads out to the airport for fuel. As we ride down to the first floor in the elevator, I tell our young woman what to expect over the next hour. That the trauma team and physician will be asking her a lot of question, drawing blood and lots of x-rays. She may also end up with a chest tube if she has a collapsed lung or blood in her chest, then an orthopedist will evaluate her for her pelvic and femur fractures. She is appreciative, and as we enter the ED and turn into the trauma room, I can't help but notice that our boss is there, talking to the charge nurse. I give her a quick up-nod as we roll the patient past her and into the trauma room, giving a verbal report to the awaiting team.

After Mike and I transfer the woman onto the ED gurney and move over all the IVs, we gather our equipment onto our gurney and roll it out into the hallway to clean it and start restocking the items we have used. As we are gathering equipment and wiping off the gurney, our boss walks up and starts asking about our call. The two of us start telling her how we landed in the snow, then as we have all our equipment together and can hear Tom on the radio, letting us know he is about three minutes out, we invite her to go with us to the roof to finish putting the ship together. As the three of us are riding up in the elevator, I start getting a funny feeling about her interest in the call or in us and finally ask, "What exactly are you getting at?" She pauses for a moment, then I ask a second question, "You never come in on night shift unless someone is in trouble. What's up?"

She smiles and chuckles as we exit the ready room, and as we start walking up to the roof, we can hear Tom shutting down the turbine engine. She then starts telling us that she's received a complaint.

"What? Who?" the two of us ask almost simultaneously, then before she can answer, I ask, "Are you talking about this call? The one we just got back from, or something else?" I am now searching my brain, trying to think of something, anything that I may be in trouble for, and in reality, I can't think of one thing. I think to myself, *Well, I guess it matters how far back she goes!*

She then tells us, "Yes, it is about this call."

Amazed, I ask, "How can that be? You were here before we were."

Holding up her hand to stop our barrage of questions, she then starts to tell us what she knows just as Tom walks up and asks, "Hey, what are you doing here? Is someone in trouble?"

"Yes, we are!" Mike says, not waiting for the boss to answer.

Now knowing she is outnumbered three to one and we are getting defensive at our patient care, she once again tries to stop us from talking, and we finally let her tell us what is going on.

"I received a call from the Plumas County Sheriff's Office. The deputy that responded to the snowmobile accident with search-and-rescue was pretty pissed off that you guys flew in and picked up the patient before he could get on scene."

"Well, that is absolutely stupid!" I say.

Mike only chuckles, then asks, "So were we just supposed to land in the parking lot or circle the scene and wait another hour for some deputy to arrive before treating our patient? You do realize that she is in critical condition, don't you?"

Knowing that the three of us are not only mad now that someone is challenging our treatment of this woman but also that the reason we are in trouble isn't from doing a bad job but from popping some deputy's ego, she then informs us that according to him, the county's policy is that the helicopter isn't to be called until the search and rescue personnel snowmobiles into the scene, make a determination if a helicopter is needed, then call the appropriate one. All three of us then answer simultaneously, "That's stupid!"

Now really mad, I can't stop and continue, "Excuse me, but I was always taught that patient care comes first, and"—I hold up one finger—"number one, we were rightfully dispatched by the ambulance crew and"—now holding up two fingers—"number two, requested to fly the road and find the woman." I then take a breath, then ask, "So what exactly did we do wrong? It's not like we swooped in and stole a patient transport from another helicopter service or the ambulance. They asked us to go look for her!"

Knowing we are in the right and the deputy is mad mainly because his ego is getting the best of him, she explains to us that she is only trying to come up with the whole story so she can do a follow-up call to explain the entire situation to him. Also, knowing that the three of us are not only confused as to why we are even having this conversation and knowing that we are all mad now, she tells us she will call the ambulance, talk to them, and then talk to the deputy and explain that we were directed to the patient and it really wouldn't have been a good thing to wait any longer before landing and helping her.

As she turns to leave us to put the helicopter back together, she knows we are upset now about what we think, that we not only did our jobs but we also did the right thing. The three of us talk about it for a while and, when we finally finish with cleaning and restocking the ship, head back down to the ED, still wondering who this Deputy Ego really is.

The rest of the evening, every time Mike and I bump into each other, we talk more about the call and keep trying to think if we really are missing something, and each time we come up with the same answer to the same question, "Would you do anything different?" And the answer keeps coming up: "No."

A couple days later, our boss catches up with us and fills us in that she talked to the Chester ambulance crew and they thought everything went well and were very happy they didn't have to ride in on snowmobiles and also added to not worry about that deputy. They have run-ins with him all the time, and in fact, he usually gets on the radio, responding from Quincy, telling the ambulance personnel to not do anything until he gets there. She then tells us that she did follow up with the deputy and tried to explain to him that the helicopter was directed to the scene by the ambulance and everything we did was totally within reason and protocol. She then goes on to tell us that he kept telling her that according to their county's search-and-rescue policy, the ambulance can't call a helicopter unless he is on scene and he will call it. She tried to explain to him that sometimes the helicopter is going to be the fastest means of not only finding someone but also extracting them out and this can save hours of time, which can be very detrimental if someone is critically injured. Then she finishes with telling us that try as she might, she couldn't convince him that we did everything correct and, in fact, the ambulance and helicopter followed not only their own policies as far as requesting aid but Nor Cal EMS's policies as well and that the sheriff's policy was only the sheriff's.

We all stand there thinking about this, and I finally ask, "So what do we do next time, hover over the patient until Deputy God arrives?"

The boss just shrugs her shoulders and tells us that she ran this by the Chester ambulance and their answer was, "Yes, sounds right." When she asked them if they had any ideas, they responded, "Yeah, do exactly what we do, ignore him." Then they added, "You can't educate him with logic. We've tried. Trust us when we say, it's all about his ego. He has to be in charge. Just do what is the best for the patient. That's what we do." She agreed with them and passed this along to us.

About then, Tom breaks into the conversation, saying, "What a dickhead."

Mike and I just shake our heads, and the boss does the same. We know she has tried her best and was put into a difficult position, as she wants the helicopter to not be stepping on anyone's toes but, at the same time, wants to do what is best for the patient. All three of us know that you can't please everyone all the time, and this is one of those cases, and it may happen again.

I would learn later that this was the same deputy that was on scene of the Strawberry Valley ("Long Night in Bi-County") incident, and unfortunately, I would have a couple more run-ins with him and his ego later on in my career.

8

SCOTTY'S

BY NOW YOU have probably figured out that in Chico, in the summer, there is always one thing you can count on—it's hot!

The next thing you can count on is that people will figure out a way to stay cool or cool themselves off during the scorching hot summer days. Working night shift, I've found things I can do during the day to stay cool are going to a movie, going to the mall, and going to the gym. All these places are air-conditioned; all you have to do is brave the heat to get there.

Most of the students who are living on Top Ramen and mac and cheese and can't afford to go to movies, the mall, or don't have a gym card can be found in one of the many swimming holes around the area. During the week, most students will make the short walk, bike, or drive to Chico's own Bidwell Park. Listed as one of the largest city parks in the United States, it contains everything from high mountain mesas to open lava flows and ends in town with many walking, running, biking, and equestrian trails to suit most adventurers. Running the entire length of the park is Big Chico Creek. As this creek runs down through the hills and lava flows, there are many great swimming holes, and any weekday will find all these spots overflowing with teenagers trying to stay cool.

But the biggest and funniest way for these students of history and political science to spend their time, especially on the weekend, is to go to Scotty's Boat Landing and float the Sacramento River. This is pretty much an all-day float down the river. The floater will be there for many different reasons, to cool off, to drink beer, to hang out with friends, or just swim.

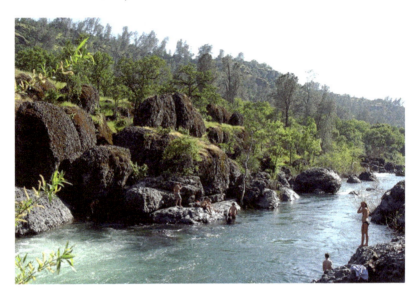

There are several problems that students, especially new students, won't know but will experience in their very first float down the river. First, they never think they need sunblock. Come on, it's 110 degrees out; you're going to be sitting in the one same position for possibly six hours, and due to your ingestion of ice-cold beer, you are not thinking things all the way through. You will get burned!

I can't tell you how many young girls I have taken care of in the emergency department over the years that would come in, arms hanging to their sides, walking like their legs won't bend, their entire back, including their butt and legs, still bright white and their entire front face, chest, abdomen, arms, and legs bright red, burnt to a crisp. Many of these girls that have just moved down from the mountains, wearing long-sleeve shirts and Wranglers, have had very little to no sun exposure, now walking in with second-degree burns and with blisters already forming on their delicate young skin. They are crying and demanding we make it better. In reality, there is very little we can do. Most of them are still carrying an alcohol load that is above the legal limit for driving, which also means we can't administer narcotics. There really isn't any cream or lotion we can put on the burnt areas. The best we can do is to maybe give them a shot to lessen the pain for the night and tell them that they will just have to survive the next week or two until all their skin sloughs off.

Occasionally, we will see different forms of trauma, usually abrasion and bruises from hitting rocks, limbs, or other tubers. Once in a while, a laceration. These are usually on the bottom of their feet from stepping on a broken beer bottle at the bottom of the river.

One of the other things the Chico State tubers have designed for their float down the river is a designated bartender. This selected individual will not only be floating the river on his tube but is also in charge of the ice chest for his or her group of tubers. One of the ways the bartender tuber has come up with to enjoy their own float with little to no attention to the ice chest is to place the ice chest, loaded with an assortment of different beers in ice, into a separate inner tube. This tube is then attached to the bartender tuber by a rope that is tied to his or her own tube. This way, they can float the river, sipping on their own brew, and have the ice chest only a short rope pull away.

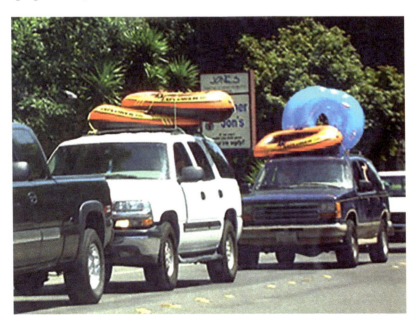

On this incredible, scorching hot day, the weather has been in the hundreds for weeks, which means by the weekend, there will be no parking anywhere near any kind of water. The closest you can park to the launching site is a good one- to two-mile hike. As our group puts into the water, the guy that has lost the toss is tying the rope not around his tube but has decided to tie it around his ankle as one of the others is securing the ice chest into the second tube. All the remaining people are lecturing him that above all things, he should not let the ice chest get lost or tip over, spilling all the beer. Our boy agrees and, before he casts off from the shore, pulls out a cold one for each of the members of his party, then they all push off from the shore and start their float down the river.

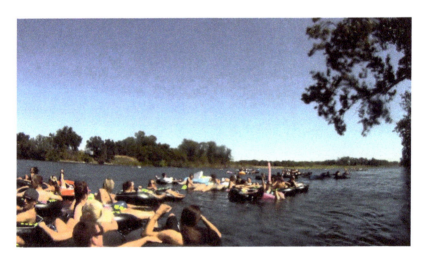

Now, a couple of hours into the float, everyone is having a good time when one of the group needs another cold one. Looking around, he doesn't see our friend the bartender and starts yelling for him. After a few minutes, the rest of the group are also yelling for him, and in disgust, they think he has floated away with another group who may have convinced him that their group is much more fun and he should ditch the first group and go with them instead. They decide to put in to shore and wait for him, as they are all in agreement that he was the last one in the float and will have to come by them eventually. As they stand in the shallows, one of the group starts getting a little concerned, thinking maybe he's had some trouble, the most common of which is a tube going flat. One of the others from the group then voices that that would be okay, as long as he doesn't spill the ice chest. As they scan the hundreds of others in the water as they pass by, one of the group notices a commotion upstream, about a quarter mile. They cannot tell what is going on, but a sudden sickness starts coming over them.

Back upstream, another group of tubers is floating down the river when one of them notices what appears to be a partially submerged ice chest. Curious, they paddle over to see if there may be some unclaimed beers for the finders. As they get to the ice chest, they can see that it has a rope on it and the rope seems to be tied to a deflated inner tube that is caught up in some heavy branches from some of the willows that grow along the shoreline. As they start pulling on the ice chest and tube, trying to claim their prize, they find a second rope that runs from the deflated tube to something under the water. As they try to pull on the rope, the current is working against them, and now three of the boys are pulling with all their might, wishing they had a pocketknife when one of them reaches down to see what the rope is caught on, thinking maybe he can untie it. As he tugs in one great pull with all his might, he can feel what he thinks is a heavy limb and suddenly is surprised to pull to the surface a tennis shoe with a foot and leg in it. Stunned at first, until he finally figures out what he is looking at, in horror, he lets go of the appendage and he falls back into his tube. Now screaming at the others, he is trying to tell them that there is a person attached to the rope. The rest of the group try and try to pull the boy up, but the current is pushing him in and under the bush. Yells and screams start passing up the series of tubers to call for help, and after a few minutes, the calls for help get back to Scotty's, and they immediately launch their boat while another calls 911.

By the time the boat reaches the yelling tubers, the rest of the first party have worked their way back to the site, now horribly worried that their friend may be what all the commotion is about. After the rescuers in the boat arrive, they start cutting away at all the foliage and pulling on the rope, and finally, with one great tug using all their might, they free the submerged student. With a second pull, they hoist him from the water, and as fast as he lands on the bottom of the boat, they start CPR. The driver of the boat throws the throttle to full, and the jet boat launches across the water back upstream to Scotty's Landing. By the time they arrive, elements from the Butte County Fire Department and an ambulance are sitting in the parking lot, and the crews are at the marina. The young man is lifted from the boat and placed on the gurney, and CPR is continued back to the ambulance and then a code 3 run is started back to Chico. Paramedics in the back are starting IVs, pushing medications, shocking his heart when appropriate, and a pair of firefighters are riding along, performing CPR.

Back at the hospital, when we receive the radio report, the ambulance crew is about five minutes out and fills us in on the status of the patient. It doesn't sound good. He had been underwater for at least forty-five minutes, a five-minute boat ride, and now the ambulance has had him for ten minutes and he is still pulseless. All in all, it has been an hour since he took his last breath, and the water he drowned in isn't considered a cold-water drowning. His chances by now of regaining any signs of life are poor, and even if he does gain a pulse, he could easily be brain-dead.

The ambulance pulls up on the dock, and the ED tech and I are there, waiting to help them unload. As we roll the patient into the trauma room, they fill us in that he still has no pulse. They did intubate him, and they are on their third round of ACLS medications. We move him over to the gurney, and the ED tech takes over the job of performing chest compressions as an RT takes over the airway, forcing oxygen down the tube into his lungs. We attach him to the cardiac monitor and take up where the paramedics have left off, pushing medications. The ED doctor is also at the bedside, talking to the paramedics as they try to determine just how long this young man has been without any signs of life. We know he is thinking of pronouncing him, as it has now been around an hour and fifteen minutes since the tube with the ice chest got hung up in the bushes and he was pulled off his tube by the current and sucked underwater by the strong current of the Sacramento River.

As the physician is now asking if any of us have any ideas, looking at the large clock on the wall to see what time to determine his death, he takes one last quick glance at the cardiac monitor, then a second glance, when the flat line that has been there for the last fifteen minutes has what appears to be a complex, a single heartbeat. Everyone is watching, thinking it may just be an agonal beat, when there's another, then another. Everyone is stunned, and the physician places his hand on the young man's groin, and his fingers are feeling for a femoral pulse when another complex appears on the screen and the physician surprisingly says, "He's got a pulse!"

Shocked, I reach down and place my fingers on his carotid artery, and sure enough, I feel a pulse. Looking up at the monitor, I watch as the rate of the complexes starts picking up and the corresponding rate of the heartbeat I feel in my fingers does the same. "Shit, who would have guessed it?" the doc says, now smiling. The rest of us get real busy now. We have other medication drips to start, trying to keep the heart going, which everyone has worked so hard at. The RT has called his department, and a ventilator has arrived. The young man is placed on it. We insert a Foley catheter into his bladder, which has a temperature probe built into it, and soon read the patient's core temp and see that, indeed, he is still fairly cold.

After about a half-hour, we have the patient fairly stabilized and, with the help of the ED tech and an ICU nurse, start up the elevator to the ICU. We enter a room and slide the young man over to the bed, and as we walk from the room, I look back and wonder what the outcome will be. Will his heart keep beating? Will he have any brain function at all? Will he have any life at all? Or will he just be a vegetable or, worse, an organ donor.

As I stand there at the door, I feel someone walk up next to me, placing a hand on my shoulder when I hear Drena's voice. "I'll keep an eye on him."

"Thanks! I'd appreciate that."

I smile at her as I turn and help the tech push the gurney back to the ED.

Over the next couple of days, I often wonder about our young drowning patient. Drena has told me he is nineteen, a student, and she had talked to several of his family who were with him at his bedside, and they all wanted to thank us for what we had done. I wasn't really sure what that was, but I have learned that families will always prefer to saying goodbye to a warm body with a pulse than a cold body in the morgue.

Three days after taking care of our young man, I'm working in the ED, taking care of a drunk in the hallway, telling him that the mop bucket is not the urinal, when I see Drena walking toward me. As she listens to my lecture to the drunk and I point out where the restroom is, she grabs me by the arm and, pulling me to the nurse's station, tells me, "I have something to tell you."

"I hope it is good news, as this night really isn't going well so far."

"Oh, trust me, you'll like this."

Now she knows she has my curiosity, and stopping at the charting area, she turns and asks, "Do you remember the young man you took care of that drowned at Scotty's?"

"Yes, I remember." Fearing that he has either been pronounced brain-dead or has passed away, I don't understand her smile when I ask, "What?"

After a pause, she answers, "Believe it or not, he is sitting up in bed in the ICU, eating a pizza."

"No way!" I say, shocked. "Are you kidding me?"

"No, really, he started coming around yesterday evening and now is totally awake and seems absolutely fine. Can you believe that?"

"No, I can't."

We talk for a while, and she knows she has cheered me up for more than likely the rest of the week. I tell her I'll try to make it up there, that I'd like to see him, and she tells me that would be a good idea.

As Drena leaves the ED, I feel like I'm on cloud nine. With a big smile on my face, I turn back to my duties, and the first thing I see is another drunk patient standing in the hallway, urinating into the mop bucket. Try as they might, none of the patients can get me down. It always feels good to be a part of saving someone's life, and as I'm standing there, watching the drunk urinating in the mop bucket, I almost feel like opening my fly and joining him. But instead, I just smile and shake my head, thinking, *What the hell! It could be worse.*

9

CHARCOAL AND EWALD

I BELIEVE ONE OF the hardest times for me in nursing school was the psych semester. I did learn a lot, and I guess that can be taken two different ways. First, there are times to be compassionate for people that are going through a crisis or have a serious mental issue or serious handicaps, and second, there are people out there that simply want an easy way out and are looking for a handout.

During our student rotations, we had to spend time in two different psych units. The first was the county mental hospital. This was a locked-down unit, and I can tell you, the people in there definitely had problems. Most of them were there because their families had given up on them and they would be on the street if they got off their medications, and the staff of doctors, nurses, psych techs, and orderlies were there really trying to help these people get back into society and lead somewhat of a productive life.

There were several different units within this facility, from group dorms to individual padded cells. One of the primary things they tried to teach these people was routine. They did the same thing every day. Get out of bed, put on your clothes, eat breakfast, stand in line to receive your medications, then before individual or group sessions, they would send them outside for some type of physical activity. Usually, this was a volleyball game. In reality, I think it was a way for the staff to see if the patients were overdosed or underdosed on their medications.

Underdosed patients would sometimes get a little too upset or borderline violent. I remember one young man that, before the game, went to the table in the common area to get his daily checkoff sheet. The staff would put new ones out every morning; the patients had to get theirs and take them with them to the different therapies, PT, meds, and sessions to have them signed off. On this day, someone had done the unspeakable and, while shuffling through the pile, looking for their own sheet, had placed this young man's back in the pile upside down. This totally threw him off, and he couldn't find his until someone helped him, then he spent the rest of the morning going around, asking each of the other patients if they had turned his sheet upside down. Then not getting the answers he wanted, he started on the staff, telling them his sheet was upside down.

I remember one of the councilors telling him, "If this is the worst thing that happens to you today, you're going to have a pretty good day!" And to this day, that is one of my favorite quotes. But for our young man, this didn't help; he needed resolution. So as we started our morning volleyball game, you could not only feel the tension building up inside of him but could also see it. He was just standing in one spot on the court, face turning red, fists clenched. Then, someone on the other side of the net hit the ball, and you could see it coming right for him. With a right hook that would have made Mohammad Ali proud, our young man returned the ball back over the net, and as it was passing over the players on the opposing side, it was still gaining altitude. Everyone on the court watched as the white ball flew overhead, then shot over the barbed wire on top of the chain-link fence, and finally came down in the parking lot, bouncing off several cars. One of the counselors then turned to the young man and, in a cool, calm voice, said, "So I'm sensing some hostility issues here." The young man, face still red, fists still clenched, just looked up and smiled with an evil smile that resembled Jack Nicholson's smile in *The Shining*.

Later that afternoon, I was asked to assist in a takedown of our man when he finally went over the edge and became violent. We had to get him down off the cabinets in his room, then hold him on the floor as a nurse gave him a shot of Haldol. We then put him into one of the padded rooms for the remainder of the day. It was amazing to watch how such a simple little thing, his sheet of paper upside down, set him off.

On another day, back on the same volleyball court, I was watching a gentleman, about fifty years old, that just seemed off. He wasn't his normal self. Usually, he would greet me, the other students, and the staff each morning with a "Good morning, how are you?" He would be in clean clothes, clean-shaven, and his hair perfectly combed. This morning, it looked as if he slept in his clothes, had not shaved, and his hair was barely pushed out of the way. When I tried to talk to him, he didn't or couldn't focus on me and just mumbled. Now, on the volleyball court, he just stood there, looking forward at nothing, slowly swaying back and forth, as if he were trying to keep his balance on a boat rocking back and forth in the sea. Then it happened, someone hit the ball over the net to him. He did see it coming but only got one arm straight out to his side, and we all watched as the ball hit him in the head. Like a giant sequoia, the man didn't take a single step to catch himself but started leaning farther to the side then, picking up speed with the help of gravity, fell to the ground, still holding his one arm out to his side as if he were signaling to turn while riding a bicycle. As the staff gathered to help him back up, one of the orderlies said, "Maybe we should cut back on his medications?"

So yes, I came to the realization that the volleyball game was just a test to see if every one of the patients was properly medicated. This was the county psych hospital, a place where there truly were people with psych and social issues that really needed help.

Then there was the Resort. This place was unbelievable to me. It housed two different types of patients. The first were adults. The only way they could be admitted was if they had medical insurance. Their primary reasons for being admitted was, they couldn't take it anymore. I learned that these people were really only there to escape reality. They obviously were well-off in their lives and only wanted a vacation. This place was so exclusive that it even had tennis and racquetball courts. And on their list of things to do during the day was thus: have breakfast served to them, schedule time on the court, and if they have time, check in with the counselor. I sat in on a couple of these sessions and decided I couldn't do it anymore. These people were trying to convince the counselors that they had problems dealing with society. Maybe it is in my upbringing, but I thought some of these people should have just received a slap across the face or a swift kick in the butt as you pushed them out the door and telling them to get in their Lexus and go back to work. Or take them over to the county facility and lock them into one of the padded rooms with a disturbed patient that was really mentally handicapped and couldn't function in society. I bet that would straighten them right up.

The second group in the Resort were minors. All the kids less than eighteen years of age had to go here. They couldn't put them in the county lockup with the really sick adults, so the Resort had a juvenile section. Once again, I could only see a game being played. These kids were having a ball, pretty much doing what they wanted and when they wanted to do it. Midway through one week, there was a new admit, a young man about fourteen. When he arrived and was placed into the group, immediately he was greeted with the high fives, hugs, and welcomes from his friends. I listened in on some of their conversation, and it was all about what they could do to find ways to be admitted back into the Resort. We were playing right into their plans. They really had no reason not to be out in society and, when discharged, tried everything they could do to get readmitted. No school, no parents, three meals a day—this was a pretty good deal for them, and they could hang out all day with their friends. I often wondered what happened to some of these young people. What happened when they turned eighteen? What road of life would they go down?

All in all, I must say I did learn a lot from both places. That there are really mentally sick people and there are really not mentally sick people but people that just want attention and know how to play the system. This I would see time and again in my career. I would really feel for the seriously mentally handicapped, knowing they are having a true emergency and need help. But then there are the ones only looking for attention.

The most common of these we would see was the female college student. Either having a bad day because she found out her boyfriend was banging her best friend or she had been out partying too much and didn't get her term paper done and was trying to come up with an excuse to tell the professor why it was late. These young women would show up at the emergency department with friends, stating, "She took a handful of pills!" Most of the time, it would be Tylenol or Motrin, and in reality, the dose they took was no more than what they would take if they were having menstrual cramps, but they would have a procession of people with them all holding their hands and the girl would be getting the attention she wanted.

Then came the hospital treatment. Just like the two different psych hospitals, you would find two distinct types of nursing treatments in the ED. First was the compassionate nurse. This nurse would hold the patient's hand, telling them, "It's okay, everything will be just fine!" Don't get me wrong, I do have compassion, but in my experience, it always seemed to me that we were feeding into the patient's need for attention, just like the young kids in the Resort, and I would see these young women repeat this scenario over and over. The problem being that as they did this, they would eventually have a psych consult and possibly be put on some type of antidepressant medication. Then they would put themselves through the same scenario, only this time take a handful of the antidepressant, say Elavil. They didn't know how bad this medication really was. I had seen these young women come in overdosed on Elavil, and it was really hard taking care of them, knowing that they would now be going through multisystem organ failure and might actually be dead in less than a week. Not at all the plan they wanted; they only wanted attention and someone holding their hand.

Next, we have the second type of ED nurse, and yes, I fit into this category. First of all, I must make a disclaimer and make it perfectly clear that yes, I do care. I want these young women to have productive lives, finish school, get married, have a family, and most of all, I want them to remember me.

I'm not going to hold their hand. I'm not going to let their friends in the room so they can continue to cry and gain sympathy. I am going to make this the worst experience in their young lives. I want them to think twice before doing this again.

CHARCOAL AND EWALD

So when a young woman comes into the ED saying, "I took a handful of pills" this sets into motion a well-rehearsed treatment plan. First of all, I tell all her escorts to go wait in the waiting room, then having the young woman alone in a room without her team of support and now only with the ED tech and myself, we have her remove all her clothing and get into a hospital gown. This not only demoralizes them a little, but the main reason is still coming. Then we ask them to drink a cupful of activated charcoal. This medication will bind with most medications that are still in their digestive system. But 99 percent of the young women will take one look or one sip of the thick, gooey, horrible-smelling, and horrible-tasting black substance and either say no or they lead you along, holding the cup to their lips, like they are sipping it but, in reality, are not. I will then point to the clock on the wall and tell them, "You have fifteen minutes. After that, I will put the charcoal into your stomach for you."

When the big hand on the clock finally reaches the fifteen-minute mark, the ED tech and I will go into the room with our arsenal of big bad overdose equipment. As the patient watches, the two of us start setting up, which includes hanging a large bag on the IV pole, filling it with 3,000cc of water or saline, and putting on waterproof gowns, gloves, and facial mask. At this point, the young women will start getting nervous and start chanting, "I will drink it, just give me a little more time." We continue to set up, telling them they've had their time and time is now of the essence, which is true, because if there really is a handful of pills in the patient's stomach, it is being dissolved and absorbed. We then place a surgical cap over their head and try to tuck as much hair into it as possible, but also knowing it is just going to come out. About the time we pull out the restraints and start tying their hands and legs to the gurney, now they are coming to the conclusion that something very unwanted is about to happen to them, and they are wishing the hand-holding nurse were on duty tonight.

Now with the patient tied to the gurney, cap and gown in place, I pull out the Ewald tube. This gastric lavage tube is a sight to behold. It is usually a 37 French, which, if you don't understand medical sizes, just hold your hand out in front of you and stick up your thumb. Yes, it is about that big. When the patient sees this thing for the first time, all kinds of bargaining starts happening. But something I learned in nursing school in the psych hospital is, psych patients can outbargain you, and most of them really have no intention of keeping their side of the bargain. Then as we are closing the door to the room, the young woman will start her struggle, and the ED tech will grab her head and try to hold it in place. I lube up the tube and, with the assistance of the tech, open the woman's mouth and start advancing it into her mouth, down her esophagus, and into her stomach. The young college student is now scared out of her mind as we tape down the tube to her face and check for placement to make sure it is really in her stomach and not her lungs. Once this is done, we attach it to the tubing on the large bag hanging over the bed and to a second one on the floor. The Ewald tube is a double-lumen tube, so you can push clear fluid down and pull dirty fluid out at the same time. We attach the lavage syringe, which is a large double syringe that will do both, push fluid into her stomach and pull the "lavaged" content out, letting it go to the collection bag on the floor. Now we start pumping the syringe and watch as clear fluid goes into the woman's stomach and also watch for what is coming out, mainly looking for any type of pill fragments. We continue this until the fluid coming out is just as clear as the fluid going in. When we reach this, we grab the charcoal in the cup that the patient has had a chance to drink themselves and suck it up into a syringe and, as promised, push it into the woman's stomach, followed by a bolus of water to flush out the tube. When we have accomplished all this, we pull the tape from the woman's face and, in one motion, pull out the large tube, which resembles pulling a large black snake out of a hole.

    At this time, both the ED tech and I step back from the gurney, as we know there is a 99.99 percent chance that the woman is now going to lean forward and puke the black goo out, covering her face, any hair that has come loose from under the cap during her struggle, and all down the front of the gown we've put on her, and by the time she is done vomiting, it is now dripping onto the floor. In essence, everything is covered in sticky, puked-up black charcoal.

CHARCOAL AND EWALD

I once asked a very experienced ED doc if there was any charcoal still left in the patient's stomach after they puked it up, and his analogy was, "If you pour paint into a can, swirl it around, pour it out, the can is still lined with paint." I could see that. It made a lot of sense to me. The lining of her stomach, esophagus, mouth, inside her nose, in her ears, and even a little extra on her skin was all going to soak the charcoal in.

Now that our young woman has willfully cooperated with the procedure, we remove the restraints from her limbs and hand her a towel to wipe her face. If you have ever been around charcoal, you will know that just wiping with a towel only smears it around, and before long, the woman's face resembles that of a Navy SEAL with a blacked-out, camouflaged face, ready for a night battle. Now is the time that I will take and have a bedside chat with our young woman. I will talk to them and discuss different options for them if they ever feel overwhelmed with life again. There are so many options out there, school nurses, counseling, or just seeking out a friend, but I make them a promise that if I see them again, they will get the same treatment and that I'm not being mean, I'm just trying to save their life.

It has been amazing to me that by this time they have gotten over their hysteria and are talking like a normal adult, and almost all of them not only thank me but promise to seek out help in the future if they need it, and all of them have promised me that not only do they never want to see me again, but they will also never be back here again.

After our bedside chat, and a little time for the charcoal to settle in, I will eventually let one of their friends in, and to see the look on their face when they walk into the room and see their friend sitting on the gurney, covered with charcoal, some still dripping from their hair, is priceless.

We also try to have one of the hospital counselors make a bedside visit to talk to the young women before we discharge them home and give them some handouts and different ideas for future needs. In the end, the young women thank us as they are leaving and have learned a valuable lesson, and I must say, I have never seen one of the young women I've treated ever come back.

10

DRIVE-UPS

IT SIMPLY AMAZES me what a person can do at times. I have seen people with arms torn from their body arguing with you that they don't need to go to the hospital, that they are just fine. The other amazing thing is what people will do simply because they don't want to get into trouble.

It isn't too uncommon while working in the Oroville Hospital ED that you may hear a horn honking, and when you look outside the ambulance door, which we always keep locked, you'll find someone lying on the ground in some state of medical need. This can range from being overdosed, hit by a car, shot, or stabbed. Either way, the person or persons that bring them to the ED want them to get help but don't want to be identified or, more importantly, be interviewed by the police. Kind of grown-ups' form of doorbell ditch.

That is Oroville; Chico, not so much. Chico is full of fun-loving college students, families with children, and a mortgage. Not as much drugs and violence, not as much, but there are still the Orovillians that make their way to the big city.

Such is the case one night when we are all hard at work, helping in the ED, thinking that we really need something exciting to happen. You also learn to be careful what you wish for. Our concentration is suddenly broken by the sounding of a car horn and someone pounding on the glass door at the ambulance entrance.

I happen to be standing at the nurse's station, close to the door, and slowly peek my head around the corner to see what all the excitement is about.

DRIVE-UPS

I don't mean to stereotype people but, if you are looking at someone that is wearing cutoff shorts, only shorts, no shirt, no shoes, dreadlocks for hair and is covered in colorless tattoos, the type usually found in most prisons, you can make a pretty good guess that something bad has or is about to happen.

As I slowly make my way away from the nurse's station toward the door, I quietly ask the secretary to call security to the ambulance entrance. I'm not sure what I am walking into but don't like the looks of it so far. As I get closer to the door, I can tell the man at the door is really wound up, pointing to the car and yelling, "Open up, open up. He needs help!" I can also see that this guy is covered in blood. As the door opens and I motion for the man to just stand there and tell me what is happening, he keeps frantically motioning for me to look into the car. Thinking this guy has driven an injured friend to the hospital for help, I bend down to look into the passenger side as I open the door. To my amazement, there is no one there. I take a quick glance into the back seat and find the same, no one. I then look further into the car and notice someone in the driver's seat. Standing back up, I ask the possibly meth-induced, excited man, "Who is it that needs help?"

Becoming more frantic, he starts shouting, "HE DOES!" now pointing at the man in the driver's seat. I nod as I then slowly make my way over to the driver's side of the car. As I walk around the front, I notice steam coming from under the hood, as it may be overheating from what I'm now betting has been a very quick drive from Oroville. I arrive at the driver's door, and as I open it, I'm greeted by another tattoo-covered individual wearing only cutoff shorts. Instantly I am also aware he is covered in blood, and there is some mess in his lap and what seems to be all over the inside of his side of the car. As I kneel down to start asking him what is going on, I can quickly make out that he is really pale. As I squat down to talk to him and to get a better look at what exactly is going on, I am suddenly speechless. I can't believe what I'm seeing and have to just take a few seconds to take it all in before reaching in to confirm my suspicions.

Now pretty sure what I'm looking at, I look up at the driver and ask, "Are these yours?" He nods as he looks back down at the mess.

I have come to the conclusion that what I'm looking at is the entire content of his bowels. I can see both large and small intestines, on his lap, on the floor, and apparently, as if this evisceration isn't bad enough, as he has been driving with all his large and small intestines on his lap, they have become entangled into and around the steering wheel of the car on the drive from Oroville and making all the tight turns through town to get to the hospital.

A couple of the other ED nurses have come out with the charge nurse and the ED tech have all joined me. The charge nurse asks me what I think, and I look up at her, shrugging my shoulders, and tell her, "You may as well activate the trauma team. Matter of fact, we may need the surgeon out here." She peeks into the car and is shocked at what she sees and, with a muffled, "Oh, shit!" hurries back into the ED.

As the ED tech kneels down alongside me, we look at the tangle of intestines, not touching anything yet, but trying to come up with a plan. One of the paramedics has joined us and asks what he can do. I tell him to go ahead and climb into the passenger side and get some oxygen and an IV going. The tech and I finally decide to start trying to unwind the intestines from the wheel. It is unbelievable how tightly they are wound into it. Some are hung up on the turn signal, and some on the gearshift. After about five minutes, the trauma surgeon has come out to see what is going on, and as he puts his head in between ours, he simply says, "Are you kidding me?" As we continue to attempt to unwind the bowels, we look up at him and ask if he has any better ideas. He studies it for a while and finally tells us to just keep doing what we are doing. The only thing he could do is to just cut them off and try to reconnect them once he has the patient in surgery, but it would be better for the patient if we can get him out in one piece.

Now, the three of us working together, we continue with the unwinding of the intestinal puzzle, at times holding several feet of intestine outside of the car to keep it out of the way as we unwind the rest. Finally, after what seems like hours but in fact is only about thirty minutes, we have succeeded in our mission; we have him untied from the car. As the three of us hold the loops of bowel, other

EMTs and paramedics help remove the patient from the car and onto the gurney. The OR crew has been standing by, watching us, and we simply hand off the patient to them and he is taken away to surgery without even stopping in the emergency department.

As I stand watching him being rolled down the hallway, I see the passenger friend standing next to the fence. I walk over to him and ask him the question that has been burning in the back of my mind. "Why did you let him drive?" Immediately he responds to my question, but not with the answer I have been looking for. "My license is suspended!"

I'm in shock. I have been thinking that maybe he doesn't know how to drive, but instead, he is totally concerned that he will be in trouble for driving on a suspended license and has told his wounded companion that he has to drive himself. Unbelievable!

As I start back into the ED, I turn to the friend and tell him, "I'll get someone to move the car for you, and by the way, the police are on their way and want to ask you some questions, so don't go anywhere." Before the doors even close, I turn back around to the sound of burning rubber as the man decides he really doesn't want to be around to be interviewed by any police officers. It is amazing that he must have forgotten about his suspended license, as he seems to be handling the car just fine. I stick my head back out of the door to watch as he speeds down the street, and just as he is about to make the corner, he nearly runs head-on into a city police car. They both come to a screeching halt, windshield to windshield. The officer jumps out and with his weapon already drawn, yells at the man to get out of the car.

I laugh as I watch the man put into handcuffs, thinking, *You know, he may have been right. He is going to be arrested for driving on a suspended license, and maybe a little more!*

As I walk back into the ED, the charge nurse asks me to write up the trauma paperwork on the patient. I think about this for a moment and, smiling, ask, "Wait a minute. He was never in the emergency department. Therefore, he was never an emergency department patient, which means he wouldn't have an ED chart. Right?"

ON THE GO

The charge nurse looks at me, thinks for about a fraction of a second, then tells me, "Nice try, just get it done."

I snap my fingers with a "Dang!" then walk into the trauma room to pull out the large trauma sheet. As I start in on the form, I can hear someone walking up behind me. I can tell they are not a nurse or ED tech, as they all have soft tennis shoes. These are more formal dress shoes, female dress shoes. I lift my head, and as I hear the shoes stop behind me, I take a slow sniff of the air, and to my pleasure, my nose fills with the pleasant perfume of the only person I know that can smell like vanilla. "Hey, Drena!" I say without turning around.

A hand lands on my shoulder, and I turn my head slightly to see her auburn eyes. "That was pretty interesting," she says.

"Yeah, you don't see that every day. Thank God!"

Drena hangs out with me as I work my way through the trauma form. As I finish, she agrees to take the copies to surgery and add them to the patient's chart. After I hand her the paperwork, I walk with her to the end of the hallway and bump the door opener for her, then watch as she continues down the hall until the doors slowly close.

Turning back around, I stare down the hallway for a moment, wondering, *Okay, what's next?*

11

911 FOLLIES

EARLY IN MY career, I started listening to the more experienced firefighters and EMTs telling their stories, and in reality, I didn't believe most of them. I would think to myself, *No one is that stupid*. Well, after forty-some years, I can honestly say, "Yes, they are!" Not only would I be impressed at times at what people would do to themselves, but more often I wondered to myself, *What were they thinking?*

To this day, I can still remember my first encounter with this dilemma. I was an EMT on the Sierraville ambulance, and the entire country was being introduced to the new nine-eleven system. You couldn't watch any TV show without some commercial on how to use it. At that time, the first introduction was, "Call nine-eleven." Everyone knew it as nine-eleven, and all fire, police, sheriff, and ambulances had new stickers to put on the side of your rigs that read thus: EMERGENCY, DIAL 911, FIRE, POLICE, MEDICAL.

EMERGENCY DIAL 911 FIRE POLICE MEDICAL

Everyone knew the nine-eleven system, and after a lot of public education, it looked as if the system was a great idea and was being accepted nationally. That is, until our one guy, that guy…you know who I'm talking about. Every system has one, someone that could screw up putting in a new light bulb or taking out the garbage. You don't understand how someone could get it wrong, but if you give this guy a job, he will screw it up.

Sure enough, that was exactly what happened to the new nine-eleven system. This guy had some type of emergency and, after much trial and failure, called the operator, by dialing 0, and telling her that he needed an ambulance. The operator, in an attempt to educate the man, asked him if he tried to call nine-eleven, and the man replied, "Yes, I tried, but look as I might, I couldn't find the eleven on my phone."

So after the nine-eleven operators started dealing with several of these special guys in different states—it seemed each state had one—they changed the nine-eleven system to the nine-one-one system. This meant that all of us that had put the 911 decals on our vehicles had to pull all of them off and put the new 9-1-1 decals on the rigs, really.

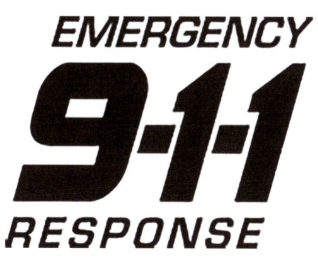

Stupid Nurse Call

After I started working at Enloe, it rapidly became more apparent that there were more people that could become confused about their health care, so much so that the emergency department kept a book of these calls and named it *Stupid Nurse Calls*. This was an accumulation of different calls from the public inquiring about medical care or what they should do about it. On slow nights, this made for really interesting reading on what new calls had been entered from the last few days.

I'll never forget one of my first calls. When I answered the phone, I was greeted by a nice female voice who introduced herself as a Chico State student, and the following conversation followed.

"Emergency department."

"Hi, my name is Shelly."

"Hi, Shelly, what can I do for you?"

"I need to make an appointment to come in and be seen."

"Well, Shelly, we don't make appointments. What exactly is it you need to be seen for?"

"I need an appointment to come in and be fitted with a diaphragm."

"A diaphragm? You mean like a vaginal diaphragm?"

"Yes, one of those. When can I come in?"

"Well, Shelly, this is a trauma center. We don't fit women for diaphragms. You said you were a Chico State student. You could go to the health center or you could make an appointment with a gynecologist in town, and I'm sure they will be glad to help you."

"You don't understand. I need to make an appointment, and I need to come in and get fitted with a diaphragm, and I need it by eight o'clock!"

After I had had a couple of years working at Enloe and seeing a couple volumes of *Stupid Nurse Calls*, a new system came out across the nation called HIPPA. It basically spelled out the privacy of patients and how EMS and nursing staff shouldn't talk about patients while having lunch in the restaurant or at the bar after work. Needless to say, the hospital administration thought that even though the stories in *Stupid Nurse Calls* weren't really patients' records, weren't in any patients' charts, and you couldn't trace any of these calls to any specific person, it was too great of a risk having the books, and they were all confiscated. Once again enforcing our knowledge that administration had no sense of humor.

Over the years, I keep looking and waiting for one of these books to show up on the shelves of the local bookstores, but I'm betting that they are stored away on some retired administrator's shelf, in their private collection, and are taken out from time to time and excerpts are read at social gatherings. Maybe bedtime stories.

12

THE NEW RECRUIT

"**I WANT YOU TO** meet Judy, our newest addition to the flight crew," says the boss. She is here to not only introduce me to the new recruit but to also make sure we don't lose her somewhere throughout the night. "Judy, this is Greg. He will be orienting you to the night shift." Now looking at me with a direct eye-to-eye, stern look, my boss adds, "And I know he will take good care of you!" I know the boss is trying to make a point not to do anything that may scare our newest team member off, like the last one. I'm sure the new flight nurse has been briefed up on the entire crew, and that may have included some very distorted rumors of night shift orientation, hazing, jokes, or a host of things that all of us night shift employees adamantly deny each and every time we are accused of such things.

I offer my hand and shake Judy's hand with a smile, then add, "Welcome to the helicopter crew! And don't believe anything you have heard about us. It is just a bunch of stories the day shift make up to scare people from working nights." Judy smiles, and even though I sense a little nervousness and her hand feels a little clammy, I think I have put her at ease. Well, maybe just a little.

"Yes, boss, I'll take good care of her, don't worry!"

I turn and, taking Judy by the arm as if we are on a prom date, escort her to come along with me as we make our way from the office, out to the elevator, to go up and do our preflight. Tom joins us and we spend the entire next half-hour quizzing Judy about her past, where she has worked, and what she likes to do. She seems like a nice and fun person; she likes to hike, water-ski, and spend time in the outdoors. She will fit in well with the rest of us.

On the ride down in the elevator, we fill Judy in on a few last things that are factually different on nights. We make sure she has a pocket flashlight, fill her in on the use of interior light in the helicopter, and when she can and cannot use them. I also tell her that sometimes we may have to leave the lights off until we are clear of the ridgeline if we are climbing out of a canyon, and it is very important to know where everything is, as we may have no lights on at all. Finally, we fill her in that if she has any questions, to simply ask. She agrees and tells us that she is really looking forward to it.

We arrive back in the ED, and after checking in, we start helping take care of different patients. I can tell Judy is a very good nurse and has an excellent mannerism with not only the patients but their families as well.

It has been a very busy evening in the ED, and finally around midnight, I ask the charge nurse if the two of us can go to lunch. She agrees, and Judy and I make our way downstairs to the cafeteria. After gathering our food, we sit at a table and I ask her why she wants to become a flight nurse. She tells me that she has always admired the crew and has read about some of the stories we have been through and thinks she wants that type of challenge for herself. She also tells me that she is amazed at the number of people that want to talk to her when they see her in her flight suit. I agree with her and tell her that I believe that 80 percent of our job is public relations. That, indeed, we spend a lot of time talking not only to patients and families but also everyone that you bump into in the hallway and elevator. I tell her, as she knows, a lot of people would love to have our job, but in reality, very few will get the chance.

About halfway through our dinner salads, our pagers start beeping. Judy and I grab our trays, and as we make our way to set them on the dumbwaiter, the audible comes over. "FlightCare, interfacility transfer (IFT), Greenville to Enloe ICU."

"This will be a great first night call for you!" I explain as we make our way to the elevator. I know she has done several flights on day orientation, and an IFT will be fairly low-key and should be fairly simple; she won't have to worry about some complicated extrication or hiking into a patient in the mountains.

We get into the elevator and pick Tom up on the first floor, then continue up to the roof. Soon we are buckled in and Tom is pulling power and lifts us off the roof. As we start climbing in altitude and heading up over the high Sierras, I notice Tom quizzing Judy a lot about airsickness and any fears of flying. Bravely she lets Tom know that she has felt quite comfortable on all the training flights and day missions she has flown. About the time we are around ten thousand feet, I look at Tom and can tell by the shit-eating look on his face that he has something planned. This also goes along with asking Judy all these questions about airsickness. It suddenly dawns on me where we are going and why we are flying a little higher than normal to get to where we are going. Tom is going to SWOOP!

Swooping was a maneuver developed during the Vietnam War. Tom was one of the special pilots chosen to insert Special Forces troops into remote locations. The normal procedure was, they would leave the base with around eight helicopters. They all looked the same, your standard Huey, all flying in a usual formation; the only difference was, only one of them had troops in it. The other seven only had the flight crews. Under the cloak of darkness, the flight of Hueys would fly a predetermined route, then when they got over the spot where the Special Forces were to be inserted, Tom would suddenly put the helicopter onto its side.

Most people don't know, but even with an engine loss, a helicopter will glide along fairly well using the spinning main rotors as an airfoil. The only way to make a helicopter drop fast is to put it on its side, therefore disabling the lift characteristics of the spinning blades. Once on its side, the helicopter will fall from the sky like a rock. Then at the last moment, he will put the helicopter back upright and pull hard on the controls, which will arrest the fall within feet of the ground. At that point, the troops will bail out of the helicopter in under one or two seconds, and he will lift the helicopter and rejoin the formation as if nothing has happened. They will then continue on their predetermined route and eventually return to base.

Now knowing what Tom has in mind for our new flight nurse, the one who says she doesn't have any kind of airsickness, I reach down and tighten my seat belt and shoulder harness as we clear the last ridge.

The Greenville Hospital sits in Indian Valley, a very beautiful spot. A natural high mountain valley surrounded by very high and very steep mountains on all sides. The usual approach to the helipad at the hospital is to clear the ridge, then start a corkscrew descent down to the helipad. We usually have to descend about three thousand feet, and this can take about five minutes, and you will usually make three or four orbits in this descent. Not tonight.

I take a quick look out my window and can see that we are about four thousand feet above the valley floor, and by the time we are directly over the hospital, which only looks to be a speck of light a long way below us, I notice we haven't started any type of descent. Looking back up at Tom, I see he has turned around, and now seeing Judy looking out the window, Tom slams the A-Star over onto its side. Instantly we are falling out of the sky. Judy is now in something just short of negative Gs, her loose seat belt barely holding her in her seat, and she is looking straight down, watching the ground raising up to connect with us. The normal sounds inside the aircraft of a whining jet engine and transmission are totally drowned out by the death scream of one flight nurse almost free-floating, trying to grab onto something, watching her life flash before her eyes. In the background of the screaming that I know would shatter glass, I can pick up the chuckles of one pilot.

I'm not sure what the liquid in the cabin is, tears of a laughing pilot, tears of a flight nurse that knows she is about to die, or urine. In reality don't know. I look out the window and can now see that the ground crew that has come out to meet us with a gurney has been watching us and, now convinced that we are falling from the sky like a meteorite and will be leaving an impact crater, have abandoned their gurney and are running for cover.

We fall the four thousand feet in about fifteen seconds. Then, just prior to hitting the ground, creating a new moon crater that they may name after us, Tom pulls back on the controls and the helicopter responds instantly, and looking out, we are only two feet above the ground. Tom then gently sets the ship down on the lawn, and I open the door. I look back at Judy. She is ghostly white, eyes as big as the crater we almost dug into the ground, a death grip on the back of the pilot's seat, the other holding a bag on the wall, her slightly oversize helmet a little crooked on her head. Tom is wiping tears from his eyes so he can see the dash to start shutting the ship down, and I just sit there, hoping Judy will have a sense of humor and get back into the helicopter with us and our patient and fly home with us. I pull my helmet off, and as I'm hooking it onto the oxygen regulator behind me, I look back at Judy just in time to see her hand traveling sideways, then *POW!* A full-on slap across my face, followed by a very upset, "THAT WAS NOT FUNNY!"

"Oh, yes, it was" comes from Tom, who has already climbed out of the aircraft, out of slapping range. I know he jumped out to give himself a head start in case she wants to run him down and beat the living shit out of him. Judy puts her face into her hands for a moment to collect her thoughts, and as I climb out, I feel a little bad for her.

"I'm sorry, I should have warned you."

Now looking up and unfastening her seat belt, she once again tells me, "That was not funny!"

I bite my cheek to keep from laughing but, at the same time, notice that she is climbing out of the ship and starting to help pull the gurney out and the medical equipment.

The ground crew has rejoined us, although I see some grass stains on their shirts from what I guess was a sudden dive behind something to protect them from the exploding helicopter when it impacted the ground. By the time we get inside the hospital and start receiving the report from the staff on our patient, Judy has totally regained her composure and is doing a great job.

We load the patient up and start our climb out of the valley, making several very wide circles, gaining altitude to clear the mountains. All the inside lights are off except the glow from the cardiac monitor. I can see Judy having a little trouble finding things but know this is all good for her, to learn to basically work by braille.

Once we clear the ridge and can see the lights of Chico in the valley a long way in the distance, Tom tells us we can now turn on the red lights. It is a welcomed event for her, as she can now see a little better. Knowing our patient is fairly stable, I start explaining a few things and showing her some tricks that she can use while working in the dark or very limited lighting. I know she is still pissed at the two of us but is asking a lot of questions and is doing really well.

We land back at Enloe, and after off-loading our patient, we ride the elevator down to the second floor as Tom goes for fuel, and roll the woman down to the ICU, and I let Judy report off to the nursing staff. We then gather our equipment and roll the gurney back into the elevator to take back to the ED so we can restock. As I'm standing there, a little afraid of what she may think of us, I look over at her without moving my head, and without looking back at me, she slugs me in the shoulder. "That was mean."

"I'm sorry, but I must say, you have handled it well, and you did much better than the last newbie."

She looks at me and thinks about asking me what happened to her, but I can see she has decided that maybe she does not want to know. By the time we push the gurney back into the ED, she is laughing and giggling. We gather up our needed equipment to clean the helicopter and restock the bag. Now, hearing the helicopter landing on the roof, we start back to the elevator and up to the roof.

As the doors open in the ready room on the roof, Tom is standing there, and Judy slugs him in the shoulder. "You pretty proud of yourself?" she asks.

Tom, still laughing, only replies, "Welcome to night shift."

The three of us quickly clean the helicopter and put the new items in the bags than head down to the ED. By the time the three of us arrive, we are all joking around, and I shake my head, thinking, *I think she will fit in well.*

We stay fairly busy the remaining early hours of the morning, and by five thirty, all of us are thinking about going home. Judy and I are sitting on a gurney in the hallway, waiting for day shift and talking about other items we will be going over the next couple of nights when our pagers start beeping.

"Enloe FlightCare, motor vehicle accident, I-5, heading two seven zero degrees, twenty miles."

"Cool," the two of us say as we push off the gurney and start toward the elevator.

We call the elevator to the first floor, and Tom arrives just as the doors open. As we ride up, I see Judy checking her watch. "You going to miss something this morning?" I ask, thinking maybe she has plans when she gets off.

"No. I was just wondering if day shift will be showing up and bump us from this flight. I haven't really had a good MVA."

Tom and I start laughing, and she only looks at us with a questioning look on her face. Finally, I speak up, telling her, "Don't worry, day shift never shows up early. They barely get here on time."

The three of us walk up and climb into the helicopter, and as we are buckling in, I ask her if she has ever gone to a scene flight on the interstate yet. She tells me no, and as we leave the hospital and head out to the west, we tell her that this is one of the most fun things we do, land on I-5. Then, to my surprise, she snaps back, "Funnier than scaring the shit out of the new flight nurses?"

I just smile and laugh.

As we approach the interstate, we make contact with the fire department and they start giving us a briefing on our landing site and then tell us that our patient is still trapped in the car. I can tell Judy is getting a little nervous about the call; not only is it on the freeway, but now there is also heavy extrication involved. "Just stick next to me, okay?" I ask, looking at her eye to eye.

She focuses on me and answers, "Like Velcro!"

Tom starts a descent to where we see the string of vehicles parked on the freeway. We can see many fire, CHP, sheriff, and ambulances, but try as I might, I can't see anything that looks like a wrecked car. "Do any of you see the accident?" I ask, scanning the area.

"No, don't see anything," they both reply.

We finish our orbit and start down to the designated spot that a firefighter is flagging us into, and then, just as we touch down, I look up and see something I have never seen before. "Oh, shit, look at that!" I'm now pointing forward out the windshield. Tom and Judy look up, and after scanning the area, they both focus in at the same time, followed by an "Oh, shit!"

Unbelievable! What we are looking at is a car, not only upside down, but also upside down completely under a semitrailer. As we exit the helicopter and approach the scene, we can see a lot of ambulance and fire personnel standing around, looking, studying. We walk up to where the ambulance paramedic and fire battalion chief are standing and ask, "Well, is there anyone still alive?"

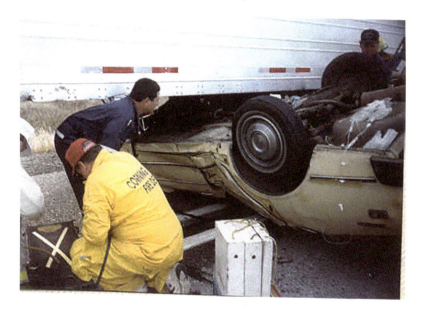

"Yes, we think there are two people in there."

"Really? And they are both still talking?"

"Yes. All they are saying is, 'Get me the hell out of here!'"

Judy and I set our gurney down and start walking around the scene to see if there is any way to get to the patients. We can see the fire department is putting the jaws together, and others are still trying to determine where to start.

I finally walk up to a CHP officer and ask, "Any idea how this happened?"

He then tells me, "There were a couple of cars in the fast lane, passing this semitruck, which was in the slow lane, when the car in the front suddenly noticed a bale of hay in their lane that had fallen off a trailer load in front of them. The first car swerved and avoided it, but the second car"—he now points at the upside-down car—"hit it, flipping it several times, then it got caught up with the semitruck and somehow slid under the trailer and was dragged for several hundred feet before the truck driver got the rig stopped."

As I listen, I shake my head, wondering, *It's amazing they are still alive.*

The battalion chief joins us and asks, "Any ideas?"

Studying the way the car is positioned under the trailer, I ask, "What if we have the truck driver back up a little?"

Everyone turns their head, looking at me with that "Are you out of your mind?" look. Then knowing they need more explanation, I continue, "No, think about it. The car is pinned up against the trailer axles. If the truck driver were back up a few feet, that may give us enough room to access this side of the car, which doesn't seem to be pinned down as much as the other side."

Now the group looks back at the car and the battalion chief starts nodding, then says, "You know, that just might work."

He then tells the group the plan, and the officer asks the truck driver to get in his truck and back up until we tell him to stop. As the driver releases the brakes and starts back, we can hear metal rubbing on metal, but incredibly, the car stays put, and the trailer axles move away from the car for about three to four feet before hanging up on something and starts dragging the car once again. We signal for the driver to stop, and now, looking in the gap between the car and trailer wheels, I can see a trail of blood running down the highway. I ask the chief if I can take a quick look in the car while he plans the extrication, and after obtaining his approval, I borrow a helmet from one of the firefighters and crawl into the space.

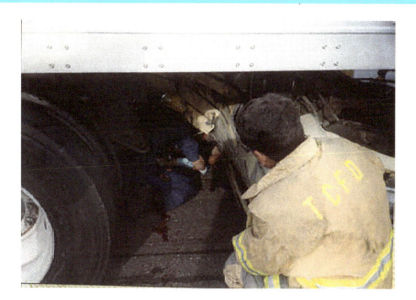

    I work my way into the space, and bending over, I can see through a small opening into the car. The two occupants have released their seat belts and are lying on the roof. As I start to talk to them, I notice the arm of the driver is fairly ripped up and broken. Looking at his position, I think it may have been outside the car when it was either rolling or being dragged under the semi. I can see a lot of blood oozing from it and ask Judy to give me some gauze and Kling to wrap it up and control the bleeding. I do what assessment I can, and knowing the fire department wants to get back to work, I tell the occupants to just sit tight, that they are in a safe place and we will get them out soon.

    I crawl out from under the trailer and join back up with Judy, the battalion chief, and the CHP officer and fill them in on what I know. I then tell Judy that from what I could see, I think there is only one critical patient, the guy with the torn-up arm, and I believe the second patient will be able to be ground-transported.

    The fire department starts in cutting the door off the car, and before long, we have access to the patients. I push Judy into the car to start stabilizing the driver while we bring out the not-so-injured passenger. After passing the passenger off to the ambulance crew, I check back with Judy and she tells me the driver is ready to take out.

Several of the firefighters have been helping her, and we start pulling the driver out on the backboard she has placed him on as she pushes from inside the overturned car. Judy finally emerges from the wreck, splotches of blood covering her flight suit, a look of concentration and professionalism on her face.

We secure the patient onto the flight gurney and, with our firefighters helping, carry him over to the awaiting helicopter. Then, just prior to climbing in, she turns, smiles, and thanks the firefighters for all their help. At that moment, I know she will fit in just fine. She not only has the skills needed but also has the professionalism to make that small gesture of thanking the fire crew. That will go a long way with them. The only thing I am still wondering is, *Does she have a sense of humor?*

We continue with treating the patient on the flight back to Chico, starting a second IV, monitoring all the equipment, and I ask Judy to give the hospital the radio report. She stumbles a little, something I would expect from someone new, but all in all, she does fine. We land and off-load the patient, and after arriving in the trauma room, she gives the trauma team a nice verbal report before we exit and start gathering replacement equipment.

The day crew is already here and asks us about the night. I choke up a little, thinking she may tell them about getting swooped, but she skips that altogether. Finally, we gather up our bags and both head out to the parking lot, talking about our night, and I finally tell her that I think she's done very well. She is really excited about the I-5 scene call, telling me that is exactly why she has wanted to be on the flight crew. I can see her excitement and try to tell her to make sure she gets some sleep today. She thanks me then, to my surprise, hauls off and slugs me in the shoulder.

I step back a little, stunned, thinking of something to say, when she speaks up. "You two scared the shit out of me with that stupid stunt!" I can only hold back a laugh, and after an eye-to-eye, burning gaze, she smiles, then laughs. The two of us laugh together, and she asks what else to expect from us. I tell her that no matter what else she may experience, it won't be as bad as the swoop. Still laughing, the two of us head out to our own cars, then I turn and yell out a final "See you tonight! Welcome to night shift!"

13

MOM AND BABY

"**OH MY GOD**, if I don't get out of here soon, I'm going to scream!" Clay tells me in passing. I can only smile as I hurry past him in the hallway, concentrating, holding an overfull urine sample that I'm trying to multitask by screwing the cap on while quickly walking to the lab. By the time I reach the lab and I'm setting the container down, my hands are soaked, and I can see that the container is now only half-full.

"Shit," I say as I set it down and look around for a paper towel to dry my hands off.

One of the lab girls sees me and yells at me to stop bringing things to her as she is already an hour behind. I look up at her and simply smile, telling her, "I'll see what I can do!" Then I add, "I'll put the CLOSED sign up," as I exit the lab and head back to the ED. Still wiping my hands and now looking at the floor, I can see a trail of splashes on the floor like bread crumbs, leading me back to my starting point. I only shake my head, knowing this is probably the other half of the urine from my overfull container and me trying to walk and screw the lid back on at the same time. *Oh, well,* I think as I bang the electric door opener on the wall and judge my walking speed to meet the now-opening door.

I immediately go back to the treatment area, where I have been helping out, and, after washing my hands in the sink, stop at the charting counter to enter some of my last observations and the treatments I have helped with on the many patients. The nurse assigned to this area is also charting, and I give her an update on what is going on as I know it, just in case I have to leave. After I finish filling her in with all my updates, she asks, if it is okay with me, that she would like to go on her lunch break. I look at her with a look of, *Really, you just stood there and listened to everything I updated you with just to tell me you are going to lunch? Next time, start with that and we won't waste any time.* Instead of entering into a conversation that will go nowhere, I take a quick look at my watch and see it is about ten thirty in the evening, and I know she usually goes to lunch around nine. "Yeah, go ahead," I tell her, then ask, pointing to two of the charts, "Is there anything I need to know about these two patients?" She fills me in that the twenty-year-old male is here for sutures for a leg laceration. It is already sewn up, and he only needs a dressing and discharge paperwork. Pointing to the next patient, she informs me the woman is here for what the patient has described as indigestion. The physician has ordered a complete cardiac workup just to rule out any heart issues before investigating a possible GI issue. I ask if she needs anything at this point, and she tells me that she should have an IV started with the blood draw, but otherwise, no, she is fine. I tell the nurse to go eat and I'll keep things going until she returns. She signs off on the charts and disappears down the hallway.

    I walk into the lady's room and introduce myself and let her know I'll be watching her until the nurse returns, and I also have to start an IV on her. The lady seems really nice and is joking with me as I do a brief exam, listening to her lungs, taking vital signs, and looking at the cardiac monitor she is attached to. I can see that she is already in a patient gown but still has her bra on. Knowing she will also be going to radiology to get a chest x-ray, I tell her that she will have to take the bra off before she goes, as the underwire and metal clips in the back will show up on the x-ray film, and jokingly I tell her that she'd have to explain to the physician why she has swallowed all those little metal clips. She laughs, and we continue our discussion while I am setting up my equipment to start the IV. As I apply a tourniquet to her arm, I know I am going to have some trouble in starting this, as this woman is fairly large. She doesn't have veins bulging from her arms, and the only place to look is in the creases at her wrist and elbow. We continue our discussion as I probe around then finally decide that I believe I have found something that resembles a vein in the fold of her elbow.

I really don't like starting IVs here as it really restricts the movement of her arm, but I also don't like poking blindly in many areas if I know I can get this going in one stick. As I prep the area, wiping it with Betadine and alcohol, she tells me that she knows they have a lot of trouble starting IVs or even drawing blood from her because of her weight problem. I tell her this is only a challenge for me. "If I can't start it, it can't be done!" We both giggle, and I tell her to please not move as I push the sharp needle through her skin. I can feel her tighten up, and as I hold her arm from moving, I slowly push the needle in a little farther, feeling for the vein.

Suddenly, I see a flash of red blood in the small sight window, and as I advance the Teflon catheter into the vein, I tell her, "I got it!" I then notice that not only is she not pulling back against my grip anymore, but her arm seems to be flaccid as well. I glance up at her and can't believe my eyes—she is totally blue, and I believe I am witnessing her last gasp of a breath. Instantly I look up at the cardiac monitor and can see she has gone into ventricular fibrillation.

"Shit!" I say, then still holding the IV that is not taped down, I yell out, "I need help! I have a code in bed 2!"

I can't leave the IV I have started before I tape it down, as we are really going to need it now. As fast as I can, I attach the IV tubing to the catheter, turn it on, and slap some tape over it to hold it in place. Three other nurses have heard my distress call and have come running to my aid. Without much discussion, one is grabbing a bag valve mask to ventilate, one is pushing the crash cart to the bedside, and the other is grabbing the defibrillation pads to attach to the patient's chest. By the time I have the IV secured, all this has been done, and I hear a "CLEAR!" from the nurse that has her finger sitting on the defibrillation button. We all raise our hands and take a step back. The nurse confirms no one is touching the patient and pushes the button. Instantly the woman's body involuntarily bounces off the bed.

We all focus on the monitor, waiting breathlessly to see if the rhythm changes from V-fib to something else that is more life-sustaining. We don't have to wait long before we see the rhythm is still V-fib and the doctor that has joined us orders us to push lidocaine and shock her again. The ED tech has also joined us and is standing on a stool, doing chest compressions, while the team performs all the other tasks. Soon the nurse with the medications yells out, "Lido in!" The other nurse that is at the defibrillator has been watching her and has already charged up the defibrillator in anticipation of delivering a second shock.

"Clear!" comes the warning for everyone to step back, and once again, the woman bounces off the gurney with the delivery of the voltage to her chest. Almost before the woman has landed back on the gurney, the ED tech is back up on his stool, getting in place to start compressions again. Just as he is about to start pushing, the ED doctor holds out his hand and yells, "Wait! I think we have a rhythm." We all study the monitor, and sure enough, there is an organized rhythm, slow at first, but picking up speed. I have my fingers on the patient's neck, searching for a pulse, and within a few seconds, I announce, "I feel a pulse."

Things really start happening quickly at this point. The doctor wants a lidocaine drip, a chest x-ray, labs drawn, an EKG, and if she doesn't start breathing soon, he will intubate her. I know the patient's bra is still on, as we never got a chance to remove it before she coded. I tell the ED tech that we need to get it off so we can get a good, clean chest x-ray, and I'll need his help to do this.

In my off-duty world, I am the king of bra straps. Early in my dating career, I had discovered a way to reach around a woman I was embracing, and with a move that resembled snapping my fingers on one hand, I could undo those little metal hooks before my partner knew what was happening. But today on my patient, she is fairly large and is wearing a bra with six or eight of those tiny metal hooks holding it in place, not the one or two of the normal-size woman I am used to. Add to this that she must have thought if she bought clothes too small for her, they would make her look skinnier. The bra seems to be sunken and embedded into the rolls of her skin. The

ON THE GO

ED tech is trying to help me roll her a little without disrupting all the other things that are happening, and I am finally able to slide my arm under her back and find the hooks. As I fumble around, trying to get a finger or two under the strap to release the hooks, I find that the more hooks I release, the more tension is being placed on the remaining hooks. After a few minutes, I'm finally down to the one last hook. I can't see what I'm doing, and I'm only going by braille. I can tell that the bra is stretched to its maximum, and I am having a real problem in trying to release that one last hook. Finally, I can feel that I believe the hook is about to release and give it one last twist. Instantly, the bra flies apart from all the tension from the patient's large frame, large breasts, and way-too-small bra. The bra comes apart almost explosively like a slingshot, and because my hand is the only other thing down there, the hook I have been fumbling with for so long slams into one of my fingers and embeds itself under my fingernail.

I let out a scream of pain and, instinctively, in a reflex move, try to pull my arm out from under the woman. I have no idea what has happened, but it feels like something hiding inside this brazier has bitten me. What I don't know is that the hook is on the other side of the patient, not my side, so as I attempt to pull my arm out from under her, it only embeds the hook farther into my finger and is now trying to separate my fingernail from the end of my finger. I can't believe what is happening to me and now know that I can't get my arm out from under the woman. I look up at the rest of the ED crew, and they are all looking at me, staring, wondering why I am screaming like a little baby.

"Something has ahold of my finger, and I cant get my hand out!" I yell.

Immediately, two of the ED nurses start laughing. The third asks, "You're kidding me, right?"

"No, I'm not!" I say as I yell in pain. "Help me! It's ripping into my finger."

The ED crew still don't believe me and I finally turn to the ED tech and tell him to help me sit her up so we can see what is going on. A second nurse steps in on my side as they see I can't help lift the patient as my arm is trapped behind the woman.

"One…two…three…lift!" the tech tells the nurse, and the two of them pull the unresponsive woman to a sitting position.

At that point, the ED doctor looks behind the woman and, after studying the situation for a few moments, starts laughing. "I don't think any of this is funny," I say.

He only laughs louder, then tells everyone, "I have never seen this before. The woman's bra is embedded under your fingernail like a fishhook." The words are barely out of his mouth, and everyone in the ED wants to look behind the woman to see the sight.

"Hey!" I yell. "Just cut the damn thing so I can have my arm back."

Now laughing almost hysterically, the ED physician pulls a pair of scissors out of his pocket and cuts off the bra on the other side of the woman. I can feel the release of the pressure and slowly pull my arm out from behind the woman, and as my hand comes into view, there is about a six-inch piece of a 38 triple-D hanging from the end of my ring finger.

I hold my hand up in front of me to study the penetrating injury and try to figure out how to remove it when I suddenly realize that the entire room is in tears, laughing. I look at them and mumble, "This is not funny. This flipping thing hurts!" At that point, I know the only sympathy I am going to get is laughter. I also know by now there is enough people around the patient that I can leave and tend to my foreign-object problem, and as I'm walking through the people, not really looking at them, but looking down, watching the blood run down my arm, I am suddenly stopped by someone in my path that doesn't seem to want to move. Without looking up, I can see the stylish shoes, dynamic legs, and skirt that can only belong to one person, Drena. I look up and see she is biting her lip, trying her hardest not to laugh, but I can also see tears welling up in her eyes as she tries not to laugh at my predicament. I stare into her eyes for a few moments then, without breaking my eye-to-eye gaze, raise my hand up between us, blood running down my arm, the cut-away portion of bra hanging from my finger. I ask, "Any ideas?" That is all it takes, and she bursts into laughter, tears starting to run down her face.

"Really, you too?" I say.

She is trying to be compassionate, but every time she looks back up at me, she only laughs harder, now leaning on me, her knees shaking, her head pressing into my chest, as if I am the only thing holding her up from falling and rolling on the floor. As she holds on to me, we both walk over to the sink, where I can place my arm under the running water to wash the blood off and get a better look as to how to pull this damn thing out. As I'm moving my hand back and forth under the water, trying to study the hook and come up with a plan, Drena finally catches her breath, and even though she is still laughing, she wants to know what she can do to help me. I instruct her to go to the supply cart and grab some hemostats.

She returns, and removing them from their packaging, I attempt to snap them onto the hook, but I'm right-handed and can't attach them correctly using my left hand. Handing them to Drena and holding my finger out to her, I tell her to snap them onto the hook. Her eyes open wider, and with a "What, me?" she stops laughing. "Yes, you. Come on, you can do this."

"I don't think so!" she replies, and the two of us enter into a discussion on why she should help me. She is defending herself, stating that she is only psych support, not nursing care, and this is definitely nursing care. Then I ask her, What kind of psych support is laughing at someone who has a foreign object embedded into their finger?

After another minute of laughter, she is finally able to speak again and asks, "Come on, when was the last time you saw someone with a bra impaled in their finger?" followed by her holding her stomach and more tears and laughter.

After much discussion, I am finally able to convince her to take the hemostats and snap them onto the bra hook. "Now what?" she asks. Studying the angle, I think the hook is under my fingernail. I tell her, "Quickly pull it out." Instantly she lets go of the clamp, and stepping back, her face no longer laughing, she blurts out, "Are you out of your mind? I'm not going to do that!"

"Oh, come on, you can do it." I hold out my hand, motioning for her to grab the clamp, then finish, "It will only take a quick jerk and it will be out."

"No way!" she says, taking another step back.

Just as I am about to explain to her that I can't do it by myself, I tell her, "Just grab the thing and I'll count one, two, three, and we will pull it out."

I can see the look of horror now on her face when an arm appears out of nowhere, and in a movement faster than a flash of lightning, it grabs the hemostat and rips the bra hook out of my finger. Wide-eyed, I stare at my finger for a moment, which is about the length of time it takes for the feeling of pain to travel up my arm and reach my brain. "GODDAAAAMMMM!" I yell out for all the patients and staff to hear. I am now cuddling my hand to my chest before placing it back under the running water. I can see the look of uncontrolled laughter on Drena's face has turned to pure horror as she watches the hook and a piece of my fingernail torn from my finger. As I stand there trying not to wet my pants, I turn to see the ED physician with a smile on his face and holding the hemostat, bra, and hook. With a bigger smile, he says, "Three!"

"What the hell?" I ask as the doctor tosses the whole bra, hook, and clamp into the trash.

Then he replies, "Just wrap it up and quit your whining!" He then turns his attention back to the patient that the team of ED nurses has now stabilized.

I look down at my finger and can see blood running down to and dripping from my elbow and turn to hold it over the sink. Looking at Drena, I ask her if she can go grab me something to put on it from the dressing cart. Still in shock from watching the thing being pulled out of my finger, she starts pulling different items from the cart, holding them up for me to see, asking, "How about this?" I know what I want but don't want to drip blood across the floor to the cart, and as I'm trying to tell her where the item is located, my pager starts beeping.

"Shit!" I say, grabbing a couple of paper towels, wrapping them around the finger as I hear, "FlightCare, scene flight, zero nine three degrees, sixteen miles. A woman in labor." I reach out to Drena as I run by and grab a small roll of gauze, leaving a dripping trail of blood as I'm running down the hall toward the elevator, now leaving her with a look of worry and concern on her face.

I arrive at the elevator to find Tom and Clay already there, and as the three of us ride up to the roof, I ask Clay to help me wrap up my finger. The two of them look at me with a puzzled look on their faces, and as Clay takes the gauze and starts wrapping it up, he asks, "What the hell happened to you?"

Looking at the both of them and knowing them and the simple fact that if they know this injury is from some old lady's bra, I'll never hear the end of it, I simply reply, "Nothing. I hooked it on something." Yeah, that'll work. I'm sure they will hear all about it in good time.

The doors to the roof open just as Clay is putting some tape over the gauze and we start up the ramp to the helicopter. The three of us buckle in and pull on our helmets, and as soon as the radio comes online, I call dispatch to find out any further information. They reply and tell us that the fire department is going to land us at the grammar school that is near the intersection of Highway 70 and Pentz Road, just past Butte College. We all know the area well and won't need the exact latitude and longitude, because the three of us drive by this school all the time. Tom lifts the helicopter from the helipad and immediately heads to the school, and within minutes of leaving Chico, we can pick up the flashing red lights of the emergency vehicles that are on scene. I have dialed in the radio frequency, and the battalion chief answers back, giving us information on our landing zone, and in no time, we are circling the school and starting to make our approach to the lawn off to the side of the school.

After we land and start walking away from the helicopter, the two of us are in a good mood, thinking that there may be a possibility of delivering a baby. We see so much trauma and tragedy that bringing someone into this world is something we really look forward to. It doesn't happen often, usually just at the back door of the ED, when a woman holds out too long in driving to the hospital and we deliver the baby in the car or the parking lot.

Just as we are walking up to the fire personnel to ask if they know anything about our patient, we can see the ambulance rounding the corner, light and sirens flashing and screaming. We also notice that it seems to be hauling ass, and this puzzles us, as most deliveries are fairly routine and Mother Nature has made sure that this is going to happen with or without you. That being said, a lot of EMS personnel don't like delivering babies and would rather haul ass to the hospital or call the helicopter to transport so they don't have to deal with it. This is exactly what we are thinking is the reason they have called us, but watching as the ambulance comes to a screeching stop, then watching as the EMT driver jumps out and is now waving and yelling for us to, "Get over here!" it just doesn't feel right.

We walk up to the back of the ambulance, and as we are setting the flight gurney down, the EMT is opening the back doors and we are shocked at what we see. Inside we can see not only the paramedic but also two other firefighters; one is ventilating the patient, and the other is doing chest compressions.

As I climb into the ambulance, trying to take the whole scene in, I ask the paramedic, "What is going on?" She tells us that according to the patient's husband, the patient is eight months pregnant, due to deliver in two weeks. She hadn't been feeling well the last couple of days and finally made an appointment to see her doctor today, which she had done. Her husband then tells the paramedic that by the time she arrived home, she was feeling worse, but the doctor had told her it is all normal for her pregnancy and she shouldn't worry. Then, approximately twenty-five minutes ago, she passed out and went into a full-body seizure.

Unbelievable! As Clay and I start our assessment, we are in shock, expecting a happy moment when we deliver a bouncing baby is quickly turning into a horrible tragedy and not just one but possibly two horrible tragedies. Our twenty-year-old expectant mother with her first child is now pulseless and not breathing. More than likely, she has been in a preeclamptic state the last couple of days when she hasn't been feeling well, and now is in full eclampsia.

ON THE GO

The paramedic tells us that she has already delivered two doses of epinephrine, two doses of lidocaine, has shocked her twice, and has basically had no change. Both Clay and I know that if the mother or child have any chance of survival, we need to get them to the hospital, NOW!

I see that the paramedic already has her airway bag out and didn't have time to intubate the mother, so I quickly snatch up the instruments and, within thirty seconds, have the tube inserted into her trachea, and I'm tying it down. Clay has finished a quick assessment and yells out the door for the fire department battalion chief to tell Tom not to shut down; we need to hot-load and get out of here.

There is nothing further to do in the ambulance, and we quickly pull her out and move her to the flight gurney, then out of the blue, while we are fastening the straps across the patient, the automatic sprinklers for the lawn come on. One of them is pointed right at us, and as all of us are trying to figure out what is happening, Clay yells out, "We have to go, now!" Not waiting to move her back onto the ambulance gurney to roll her to the helicopter, we all carry her at a fast walk across the lawn, getting hit by different streams of water. All the time we are ventilating her and one of the firefighters continues to do chest compressions.

As we approach the still-running helicopter, I can see it is also getting hit by several streams of water, one of which has shot through the door I have left open and is not only soaking everything inside the ship but Tom as well. As we reach the running helicopter, Tom is yelling at us to just get in so we can get out of here. It seems that we just throw the flight gurney into the helicopter, and somehow it lands correctly and has locked into place. I continue to squeeze the bag, forcing oxygen into her lungs, and the firefighter who is doing CPR is now standing on the helicopter step while Clay gets into his seat and takes over. As I yell at one of the firefighters to take over the ventilations, a stream of water soaks my back. The firefighter takes over the bag, and I quickly step to the back of the ship, open the rear compartment, and turn on the oxygen. I then jump into my seat, and before I can plug in my helmet, another stream of water hits me right in the face. I slam the door closed, stopping the stream of water, then attach the oxygen tubing to the regulator on the wall and crank it up to full. Clay has already attached all the cardiac monitor leads and defibrillation pads and then kneels down to start compressions. At that point, I take over the ventilation bag and wave the ambulance and fire personnel to step back out of the way. Tom has been watching all this, and before the ground crews are completely out of the way, he is already pulling up on the collective, and in a maneuver that I'm sure he learned in Vietnam, the helicopter has turned. With the nose only two or three feet above the grass, tail almost straight up, we are picking up speed as if a rocket has been lit and we have been fired off at the speed of sound. Then, just before reaching the tree line, he pulls back up on the cyclic and clears the tops of the trees by inches. I'm sure those on the ground are all still watching us and can see leaves falling from the trees, settling to the ground.

Inside the helicopter, we are working feverishly, pushing drugs, shocking her heart, doing chest compressions, ventilating all the time—all this while slipping on the wet floor. Sweat and water are both rolling down our faces from under the brims of our helmets. There is very little conversation as we both know what has to be done; we also know the longer our mother goes without a pulse, the lower the chances are for her to survive. We also know that we must give our young mother every chance at life and we must continue to circulate oxygen-enriched blood to reach her fetus if it is going to have any chance of survival. We know we are dealing with not one but two lives, knowing the only cure for eclampsia is to remove the baby and the only chance the baby has is to do an emergency C-section.

As we clear the ridge and I can see Chico approaching fast, I key up the microphone and give a very quick report to the physician on the base radio.

"FlightCare is en route with CPR in progress of a twenty-year-old, first-pregnancy, eight-and-a-half-month-gestation female who was found in status seizures and no seizure history. We are on our third round of ACLS, and she is still in V-fib. Recommend having an OB-GYN and pediatrician standing by. Our ETA is less than five minutes!"

I hope they get the hidden message that we believe that our only chance of saving either the mother or baby is an emergency C-section on arrival in the OR or the emergency department.

Somehow, Clay and I have been able to keep up on all the drug administration and defibrillation along with doing chest compressions and ventilation. I suddenly notice that the helicopter is making a banking turn to the right, and with a quick glance out the window, I can see that Tom is coming into the helipad at a very fast speed. Before we are over the rooftop, he is already turning sideways, and because of the door being on my side, we seem to come to a sliding stop, right in front of the receiving team. I quickly slide the door back and step out just as the ground crew walks up with the gurney. The woman is pulled out, and immediately, one of the techs steps up on the lower rail of the gurney and starts chest compressions. We are out of the ship in under fifteen seconds and rolling down the ramp to the waiting elevator. As we enter, Clay and I are still trying to push medications and keep up with everything we are doing. Neither one of us has taken off our flight helmets, and as we are almost jogging down the hallway into the trauma room, we can see the look of apprehension and fear in the faces of the team of doctors, nurses, and lab and x-ray techs.

Most of the team members are parents, have been through a pregnancy, or have children. They know this has been one of their biggest fears during that time, and they are all empathetic. They look at this young woman who is just starting her family, starting married life, and planning on raising children. This isn't some drug deal gone wrong, or a DUI patient; this could easily have been anyone of them.

We barely get the woman transferred over to the emergency gurney, and the OB doctor is making an incision across the woman's lower abdomen with a scalpel. In less time than it takes me to take my helmet off, I can see him pulling the small infant out of the woman's abdomen. He then turns and sets it down onto a delivery cart that the labor-and-delivery nurses have brought down with them. There is now a pediatrician at the cart, and between himself, two L&D nurses, and one ED nurse, they start CPR on the baby and are starting resuscitation efforts. I look back at the woman and see the emergency department team working as hard as they can, attaching monitors, pushing medications, shocking, assessing. The room is filled with people shouting loud orders back and forth from both of the teams, the mother's and the infant's.

I try to help out where I can, sometimes running medications to both of the teams. Then, after about fifteen minutes, the emergency room doctor, holding his fingers on the woman's neck, searching for any signs of a pulse, asks the tech to stop CPR. He looks at the monitor and only sees a flat, straight line. Removing his hand, he steps back and says, "That's it, we're done. There's nothing else we can do."

I can feel a lump swelling up in my throat but instantly turn my attention to the team working on the infant. I can see the baby through the maze of people working on it and can make out it is a baby boy but can also see it is not moving and it is totally blue. Within a minute of stopping CPR on the mother, the pediatrician, raising his hands and placing them on the hand of the nurse doing compressions on the small boy's chest, says, "You can stop. He's gone."

The lump in my throat has now moved up to my eyes, and the whole room becomes blurry as I feel tears now joining the sweat running down my face. I can say nothing. Wiping my eyes, I can see several of the people in the room openly crying. I feel a hand on my shoulder, and without turning, I reach up and place mine on hers. I know it's Drena without turning around to look at her. I feel her press herself against me, and I can hear her crying.

After a few minutes, we both take a deep breath and release our grip on each other. I look across the room and can see others still holding on to one another. I turn to the sink, and after turning the water on, I place both hands together until they are full, then dunk my face into the water cupped in my hands. The cold water feels good, and I repeat the procedure, running my hands up over my head to help wash some of the sweat off and moisten my hair to help me cool off. Feeling a nudge, I look to see that Drena has brought me a towel. I nod, taking the towel, then wipe my dripping face. Then I wrap it around my neck. Placing a hand on my back once again, she asks, "How did you get so wet?" Pausing for a few seconds, thinking about the sprinklers, I just tell her, "Long story. I'll tell you about it later." With a questioning look on her face, she turns to leave the room and starts with her job of contacting the family.

As the room slowly empties out, I know I'm going to be asked by the ED nurse to help out with the two patients. We will need to prepare them both to take them downstairs to the hospital morgue. It is not a fun task, but I also feel compelled to help as much as I can. I know Drena is going to have to deal with the husband and any other family that may be showing up and will eventually take them downstairs to let them have a moment alone with the woman and baby. I simply can't imagine what the husband will go through, and in reality, I don't want to. This isn't a crime scene, so I know I can clean up the woman as much as possible, and after placing clean linen on the gurney and over her, I make a point of leaving her hands easily accessible so a family member can hold one without reaching under the blanket. The last thing I would want is for them to pull back the blanket, looking for a hand and seeing the open abdomen where the baby was taken out.

Finally cleaned up, we have called for a very special gurney always referred to as the picnic table. It is a special gurney that you can put a corpse on then lower and has a false top that you then make up to look like an empty gurney; that way, as you are pushing a body down the hallways, or in the elevator, everyone simply thinks you have an empty gurney. A pretty cool idea, if I do say so myself.

When the picnic table arrives, we move the woman onto it and lower it. We then place the baby, wrapped in a blanket, on the mother's chest, then cover the two of them with the top and make the sheets up to look like an empty bed. The ED tech has agreed to assist the SWAT nurse in taking the gurney downstairs, and as they are leaving the trauma room, I place a hand on the gurney one last time, feeling a loss and wishing I could have done more.

The tech pushes the gurney out of the room, makes the turn, and starts down the hallway toward the elevator. I watch as he is passing people in the hallway on gurneys in the gurney garage, nurses at their bedsides, everyone totally oblivious to what is being wheeled by them, the death of an entire young family. I know the husband will be totally decimated. The parents of the young woman will also not understand. Their lives have been changed forever. Sometimes I just want to scream as I listen to someone complaining that they need another Vicodin prescription for their migraine, knowing that an entire family has been destroyed. I watch the door close at the end of the hallway, and turning back to the trauma room, I start cleaning the room, getting it ready for the next disaster that will show up.

14

HIGHWAY 70 RESCUE

"**SO WHERE EXACTLY** are we going?" Clay asks.

I'm looking out the window, enjoying the view as we fly over the mountains, headed to a location along Highway 70, a road I have been driving since before I've had a driver's license.

I key up the intercom and answer him, "I believe we are landing at one of the wide areas along the highway near some of the railroad bridges."

The call has come in as an injured hiker, and we have been requested by the local ambulance to try to find him. I know they don't want to go hiking. The hills in the Feather River Canyon are very steep, and most areas are almost inaccessible. If we can spot the hiker from the air, we may be able to set down and pick him up. I know that during the summer, driving the canyon, you see cars and trucks parked all along the road. People are out enjoying the area, fishing in the river, swimming, and hiking in the hills or just out for a drive. You also see different motorcycle clubs driving the canyon, making a circular trip that can take them to Quincy, up to Lake Almanor, down to Red Bluff, then returning to Chico. It is an all-day ride, but extremely enjoyable.

We finally crest the hill and start into the canyon. We don't drop too low too fast as there are many power lines crisscrossing the river and road running from many of the different hydroelectric dams that cross the river. I key up the radio and call the ambulance, and they answer almost immediately. As they are talking, I can hear the distinct sounds of rotor blades in the background. Knowing that is probably the sound coming off our rotor blades, all three of us look down out of the windows, and Tom banks the ship over a little to improve his view. "There they are!" he says and starts banking the ship even harder and enters into a high recon of the area so we can take a moment to look for any power lines nearby. The three of us start calling out different lines we each see out of our own respective windows, and after a few seconds, we all stare at one another and laugh. There is so much information that altogether it makes no sense. We can each see lines and don't know if we are looking at the same ones or different ones. We decide to approach it differently, and Tom says he is going to start a slow approach to the landing zone, which appears to be a wide spot just off the highway. This time, I have my door open, looking out to the front and under the ship, and Clay is doing the same on his side.

We talk Tom down and set down at the LZ without any problems. I tell Tom to keep the ship running and I'll go talk to the ambulance crew and see what they want us to do. He gives me a thumbs-up, and I unplug my helmet and walk away from the running helicopter and up to the ambulance crew. There is another person with them, and he starts filling me in that he and his buddies were hiking to a fishing spot they know up the hill. Now as he points up a small canyon, I can see a creek running down a very steep drainage and entering the main river. I ask the man, "So if I understand you correctly, if we follow that creek, we will find your friend?"

"Yes, that is correct. He is about two to three miles up there, and another friend of ours is with him."

Now understanding where we are going to have to look, I ask about what kind of injury he has, and he tells me that he fell and his leg was pinned in some rocks and they think it is broken. He has no other injuries but can't walk at all.

I thank him for the information and tell the man and the ambulance crew that we will go ahead, fly the drainage, and try to locate him. Agreed, I turn and walk back to the helicopter, and after I buckle in and plug my helmet back in, I tell Tom and Clay what I know. Tom pulls power and starts out over the road, and we know the first part of searching the drainage will be a little tricky, as there is a set of large, very-high-voltage power lines crossing it. I tell him that we have a couple of miles to go before we start looking, and this helps as he lifts the ship almost vertical until the power lines are right out the front window, then we fly over them and descend a little. I have my door open and have turned sideways in my seat so I have a better view in front and under the ship as we fly along. With the tall timber and thick undergrowth, it could be almost impossible to spot the two men without some type of aide.

As we are now flying along, slowly moving up the drainage, Tom is also having to climb, as this area is incredibly steep. I can see that the creek running down the drainage has many waterfalls as it works its way down the hill. As we follow a small bend in the creek and I'm looking down through the foliage, I suddenly spot some movement. "Wait, stop!" Tom pulls back on the controls and brings the ship into a hover, and I ask him to back up just a little. Then I say, "Stop!" Looking down, I can see a twentyish-year-old male waving what appears to be a red shirt frantically. "I think this is it," I tell the crew in the intercom. I then start looking for an area to land, and it really doesn't look good—it is so thick and overgrown that I don't know if we are going to be able to set down anywhere close by. Then Tom speaks up, telling us that there is a very large granite boulder in front of him and he may be able to get close enough to it to let one of us out. As he tells us this, I look out the front window and can see the boulder he is talking about. It is sticking out of the hillside and is about forty feet high, but from the angle I'm looking at it, I think the canyon is too narrow for the rotor blades. I voice my concern to him about this, then we decide to fly above it and make a down-canyon approach and try to get to the large rock.

As Tom pulls out and is making a circle and starting to slowly approach the boulder, I am now not only watching below us, knowing we have to fly over the trees before we can start our descent, but also having to watch the sides as we are getting closer and closer to the trees with the tips of the rotors. Clay is doing the same on his side, and just as the tail rotor clears the last tree and we start to drop almost straight down to the large boulder, Clay speaks up and tells Tom to slide over to my side about three feet. Watching the tips of the rotors on my side, I watch as they get closer and closer to the large pine trees before I finally say, "Stop!" We enter into a hover, and looking below us, I can see that we are still about ten feet above the boulder. I tell both Clay and Tom, "We still have about ten feet to drop, but we are now only about two feet from the trees on my side."

"Yeah, we are about the same on my side," Clay adds.

Then all three of us pretty much say at the same time, "This isn't going to work."

Tom pulls power and lifts the ship up a few feet before we nose over and fly down out of the drainage.

"Now what?"

I know Clay and I are thinking the same thing, that we may have to hike up the incredibly steep drainage to the injured hiker and then somehow get him out, when Tom throws out an idea. "What if we call the sheriff's helicopter? It is a lot smaller and may be able to land on the rock."

"Great idea," I say, and knowing we can't get out on the radio to Chico while in the canyon, we radio the ambulance that we are going to fly up to an altitude so we can call our dispatch and then we will be back down to land and fill them in on our plan. They acknowledge, and we make a couple of circles, gaining altitude until we can finally contact our dispatch.

Tom tells them to call and see if the Butte County sheriff's helicopter is available and gives them the coordinates of where he needs to come to meet up with us. We stay aloft for a few minutes until they get back to us and confirm that the helicopter is available, is already in the air, and will start up to our area. It has an ETA of about twenty minutes. We acknowledge, and Tom starts back down to the landing spot along the highway.

After landing, we fill in the ambulance crew and the sheriff deputy on what our plan B is. That we will fly back up the drainage in the smaller helicopter, land on the boulder, and somehow get the hiker into the smaller ship, then bring him back here, transfer him into our helicopter, and take him to Chico. Everyone is in agreement that this would be the best plan, and all of us know that no one wants to hike up to where he is.

As we are waiting, I fill in the one hiker that has hiked out on what is going on, then I have to ask him, Why do they go camping and fishing here? The climb is incredibly steep. He tells us that he and his buddies have been hiking and fishing that stream since they were kids and that the fishing is really incredible, but the main reason for this is that it is very difficult to get to and that in itself is a major deterrent to the normal angler that pretty much wants to just fish from the roadside. I agree, and thinking back to my childhood, I know exactly what he is talking about. There were a few places my friends and I would hike to that very few people would ever try to get to, and this was what made those spots special.

As we are talking about great secret fishing locations, we have almost forgotten about our stranded patient, still up in the forest, more than likely wondering, *Where did those guys go?* and *What now?* Then we are brought back to reality when we start picking up the sound of rotor blades from the Hughes 500.

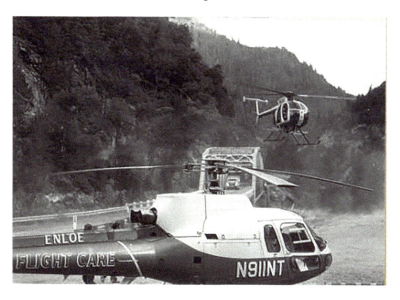

The Hughes 500 is an incredible helicopter. It truly fits the description of "eggbeater." It not only is shaped like an egg, but with its five-blade main rotor system, it does not have the typical *whop whop whop* of the bigger helicopters with their two- and three-blade rotor systems but sounds more like a very large appliance. It is extremely maneuverable and incredibly fast. We all watch as the small helicopter makes its approach and sets down in the dirt next to ours. As I take in the scene, it is funny to see how having the 500 parked next to the A-Star makes our Enloe ship look like a giant.

The pilot shuts down the Hughes, and after the rotors stop spinning, he exits, and we fill him in on our plan. Knowing we would like to take a stokes litter as we will probably have to carry the patient to the landing spot, the Hughes pilot walks to the rear compartment and, with a flip of his wrist, releases the seats and pulls them out. I am very impressed at how fast this is coming together, and seeing that the Hughes has already had all the doors removed for the summer, we slide the litter into the rear, placing it on the floor.

Not really liking what I see as far as how someone riding in the rear is going to have to wear a seat belt, I jump into the front seat. Clay stands back and studies the rear of the helicopter for a moment, then throwing the first-out bag in, he sets it in the stokes against the rear of the bulkhead, sits on it, and is then able to fasten a seat belt. As the pilot is starting up the engine, I plug in my helmet and I start filling him in on what we think will work as our landing zone.

Now with the engine at full speed, the pilot pulls up on the collective and we lift from the side of the highway. We climb up and over the power line, and I start pointing to where I believe the large granite rock is, and in no time, it comes into view. The pilot circles it a couple of times and then starts in on his approach. The smaller helicopter with its smaller rotor blades has no trouble at all descending through the trees and onto the boulder. The pilot tells us that he will keep it running for a few minutes until we are sure this will work. Clay exits the ship, and as we are pulling out our equipment and now looking over the side of the boulder, we both come to the conclusion that it isn't going to be a problem getting to the patient, as it is all downhill, but it is going to be a task getting him back up the hill and especially up the side of the boulder to the helicopter. We finally decide that we will need some rope to get this done. I lean into the ship and tell the pilot that he needs to go back and get some rope and ask if he wants one of us to go with him, and he tells me no. After making the first landing here, he feels comfortable enough and will be right back.

Both Clay and I climb down off the boulder with our gear, and when we are clear, the pilot takes off and heads back to the highway for the needed rope. Clay and I then start climbing down through the foliage and find the patient about a hundred yards from the boulder that we have landed on. As we start assessing him, he and his friend can't thank us enough for coming back for them. After we aborted our first landing attempt with the A-Star and left, they thought they were going to have to spend the night. The friend also thought that he might have to hike out, leaving his injured friend, as he now didn't know what was going on and really didn't want to have to make the climb back up here again.

We find that our patient does seem to have a broken leg, and after splinting it, we start discussing how we are going to get him up to where the helicopter will be landing and tell the friend that it is going to take all four of us to get this done. At the same time, we hear the Hughes coming back, and in no time, he is making his approach and lands once again on the boulder. This time, he shuts the helicopter down, and by the time he is out of the ship, we have already placed our patient into the stokes, and with the help of his friend, the three of us have already carried him up the drainage to the bottom of the boulder. The pilot is now looking over the edge and holding the rope, asking us what we would like him to do. We ask him to toss one end down to us, and after he does, we tie it off to the stokes, then as I look up the side of the boulder, it becomes very apparent that the pilot isn't going to be able to pull the patient up to the top by himself. Clay decides to stay with the patient and will try to guide the stokes up as far as he can while the pilot, the remaining friend, and I pull him up the face of the rock.

The friend and I climb up the side of the very steep boulder and, when we get to the top, fill in the pilot on what our plan is. All agreed, we yell down to Clay that we are ready, and he yells back, "Go ahead!" The three of us start pulling up on the rope and feel it tighten up against the load of the stokes litter. At the same time, Clay has stepped away from the boulder and, hanging on to a piece of the rope that we have left as a tag line, tries to keep the stokes away from the boulder as much as possible so it will not hang up. The problem is, he is only one guy, and he is having a lot of trouble pulling against the three of us. His feet are sliding, and he is steadily losing ground. But that issue isn't as bad as the next problem—he is running out of rope to hold the stokes straight and away from the boulder and starts yelling at the three of us, "Stop for a minute!" But what he doesn't know is, we have taken a loop around one of the helicopter's skids, and with every, "One, two, three, PULL!" one of us tightens the rope up on the skid. With all the chanting, none of us can hear Clay yelling at us, and as he is sliding closer and closer to the boulder, the three of us, knowing our end of the plan is working, pull harder and harder until Clay only has the last six inches of rope and we three are pulling him off the ground. Then, with a, "Well, shit!" he lets go of the tag line at about the same time as the three of us give one large manly pull.

The stokes jumps in the air, then slams against the side of the boulder, and the three of us on the top almost loose our footing and grip on the rope. Fortunately, we do have the rope hitched around the skid, and the pilot, who has ahold of the end, is able to quickly tighten the half-hitch and stop the stokes from falling back down the rock face and landing on Clay.

The friend and I both regain our footing, and looking over the edge of the boulder, I can see the stokes with the patient in it just as Clay backs away, looking up at us. Without saying a word, I give him a hands-up-to-my-side, the universal sign for, "What the hell?" and he only does the same.

Clay then gathers up the first-out bag and any other items he has out as the three of us on the boulder finish pulling the patient up onto the boulder and set him down next to the helicopter. As I start a conversation with him about his ride up the rock face, not asking about the part where he slammed into it, Clay makes his way around the side of the boulder and joins up with us. The pilot then tells us how he would like to load the stokes into the ship, and after securing it, I step back and notice that it is sticking out each side about six inches. I know everyone else can see the same thing as I, and knowing it is only going to be about a two-minute ride down to the A-Star, we load the rest of our bags.

ON THE GO

Now that we are ready to go, Clay then speaks up, asking the pilot, "Are you going to be able to take all of us?" The pilot then tells us that no, he will be able to take the patient and the two of us, but not only is Clay going to have to straddle the stokes in the rear, he will either have to come back for the friend or he will have to hike out. The friend only smiles and tells us that he has no problem hiking out; it is all downhill, and he needs to stop and grab all their gear anyway. He does ask us to tell his other friend not to leave him, that he should be out to the highway in a couple of hours.

We agree and shake hands with the friend, and he leans into the helicopter, tapping his buddy on the shoulder, telling him that he will gather his gear and catch up with him eventually. He then turns and starts off the side of the boulder and down the drainage to where they have left their gear. I help Clay into the rear of the Hughes, and somehow he is able to put one leg on one side of the stokes, one knee inside of the stokes along the side of the patient, then fasten a seat belt around his midtorso. It doesn't look as if it would pass any OSHA inspection, but it should keep him from flying out of the open cabin. I climb back into the other front seat as the pilot is starting up the ship, and with a "Ready!" and thumbs-up from the two of us, we lift off the rock and start down the drainage.

As we lift over the power lines and start down to the highway, I look out the open door and can see that the same people still seem to be there, and when we come in, the downwash from the rotor blades kicks up a cloud of dust, covering everyone.

After we land, I exit the ship along with the pilot, who has decided not to shut down and help Clay get out and hand the bags to Tom to take to our ship.

With the help of Tom, the pilot, and the ambulance crew that have stayed, we pull the stokes out and carry it over to the FlightCare gurney, which is lying on the ground. We set the stokes down next to it, and after we unstrap the patient, he moves over under his own power to our gurney with very little of our help. We had already given him some morphine before we left the hillside, and he is still doing well. We slide the gurney into the A-Star and, after thanking everyone, climb in, strap in, and Tom starts up the engine.

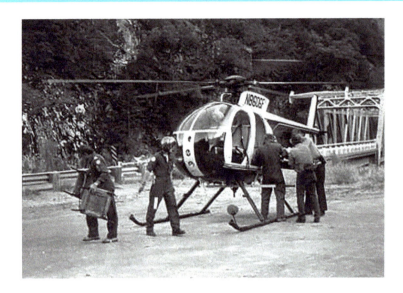

As we lift and climb out of the canyon, Tom asks us how the trip went, and looking at Clay, I start laughing and ask him, "Why did you let go of the rope?" Laughing himself, he then tells me that he had come to the end of the rope and had to let go. I then tell him how the three of us had landed on our butts when he did, and thank God we had the rope half-hitched around the helicopter skid.

The three of us laugh the rest of the way to Chico, and as we enter into final approach, a quick glance out the window and I see that the sun is just setting over the hills to the west.

When we touch down and open the door, we are hit with a blast of heat from the 115 degrees of the valley and wonder how we can go back up into the hills, where it is a very pleasant 80 degrees.

Clay and I depart the helicopter, and as we roll the patient down the ramp and into the elevator, Tom is lifting and heading out to the airport for fuel. As the doors of the elevator open, we step into the air-conditioning, pulling off our helmets, and tell the patient, "Welcome to Enloe." We then fill him in on what to expect next and that eventually an orthopedic doctor will come and evaluate him. We have decided to not make him a trauma activation, as it seems that he just has the isolated injury to his leg, so the charge nurse has us unload him into the cast room. After doing this, I pull the gurney out into the hallway to start restocking it, while Clay writes up the paperwork. As I am wiping the gurney down, a voice catches my attention from behind me.

"Are you having fun?"

I turn and smile at Drena, telling her, "Yes, we actually had a great time. The weather was great, we went for a ride in someone else's helicopter, went mountain climbing, and I fell on my butt once."

She then bends over to her side in an effort to look at the back side of my flight suit, telling me, "Well, I hope you didn't bruise anything." I tell her that I believe I am just fine, then start telling her about the rescue and that she may want to go in and talk to our patient, that he may want her to get ahold of some of his family.

We talk for a few more minutes when I hear Tom calling me on the radio, and knowing I have to go upstairs, Drena tells me to be careful and she'll catch up with me later.

After riding up in the elevator and cleaning out the inside of the helicopter, I start the task of replacing all the used equipment. At the same time, I can feel the heat of the day cooling off as the sun is now down. All around me, I can hear the sounds of the city streets and smile as I think to myself, *Okay, what's next?*

Two weeks after our rescue of the hiker up Rock Creek, our friend, the pilot in the sheriff's helicopter was flying a patrol when he sustained a complete tail rotor failure. Being the quality of pilot he is, he managed to get the helicopter down with what little control he still had. The Hughes 500 hit the ground fairly hard and was totaled, but the pilot only received moderate injuries and eventually returned to work.

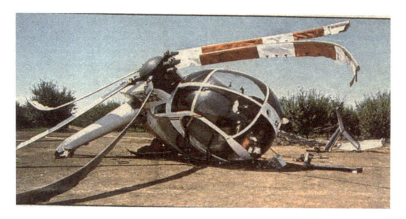

15

HORSING AROUND

"**I REALLY HOPE I'M** not going to be late for work!" I mumble, looking at Joe, my horse. It was such a nice day out when I awoke in the middle of the afternoon following my night shift that I decided to go grab Joe, throw the saddle on him, and go for a ride in the park.

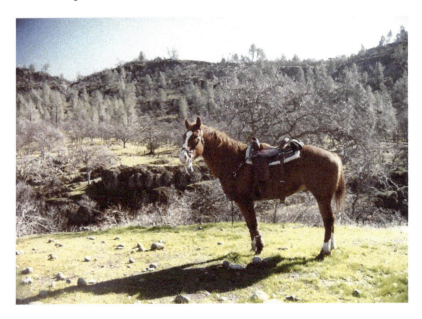

It is about five days into my six-day stretch, and I have decided, instead of the normal routine of going for a run, then a workout in the gym, I'd go for a ride and exercise my horse. We have ridden the upper trail in the park and are taking a moment to look over the edge of the mesa down into the park and the city about five miles away. From our vantage point, we can also see the creek and all of its swimming holes, and they seem to be filled with college students lying on rocks or swimming, trying to beat the heat. As I look at my watch and mount back up, I can see that it just might be a horse race to get back to the stable, unsaddle Joe, put him away, get back to my apartment, shower, and get to work on time. Looking back at Joe, I tell him, "Well, pal, looks like we are going to have to take the shortcut, and it's all about you now." He seems to acknowledge my pep talk as I head him off the side of the bluff on a very narrow trail that I know of. Most of it is so steep that Joe is sitting down on his rear and sliding. Knowing this, I loosen up on the reins and give him total control of his head and let him pick his own way down the hill. He knows where he is going, and he also knows it is time to get back. When we reach the bottom of the hill, Joe breaks into a gentle lope, and following the lower trail, he seems to enjoying the wind in his hair.

We pass a few hikers, who gladly step off the trail to let us pass, only watching in awe as the large sorrel gelding gracefully passes them by. I nod to them for giving us the right-of-way and continue to lope along the trail until we are at the pavement that we have to cross to enter the stable. As we slow to a walk, I can see that Joe is a little sweaty and, looking at my watch once again, think I have just enough time to hose him down. I toss the saddle into the back of the truck, and as Joe stands there, I douse him with water from the hose. He seems to enjoy the cooling it brings to him. I also know that there is no point in wiping him down because as soon as I turn him loose into his stall, he will lie down and roll. And as I am latching his gate, that is indeed exactly what he does, and I smile as he stands up and shakes. Even though a cloud of dust comes off, he is still covered in dirt and horse manure and seems to be happy about it. I just smile and shake my head as I toss the halter into the back of the truck and, not taking the time to remove my spurs, start the truck and let the rowels roll on the floor as I shift gears, heading across town, back to the apartment.

By the time I reach the apartment door, I am already pulling clothes off, kicking my boots and spurs off, leaving a trail of clothing from the front door all the way into the shower. I waste little time, as I only wash my hair. A quick wipe-down with some soap, and I'm out and into my room, jumping into the lower half of my flight suit. By the time I reach the hospital, I only have a couple of minutes to spare. As I am pulling into the parking lot, I notice someone on the ambulance ramp waving at me. I know this means there is a flight and the day crew doesn't want to go. I decide I don't have time to look around for a parking spot, so I aim the truck into a parking spot marked AMBULANCE PARKING ONLY and have the key shut off and out of the ignition before the truck comes to a stop, letting it coast with the clutch pushed in. When I know it is in far enough, I dump the clutch and the truck bucks to a stop. I jump out, grabbing my flight bag, and start running across the street, knowing I am quite a sight; my flight suit is on only half-on, with the sleeves tied around my waist, T-shirt on, boots on, but not zipped, and my hair is still dripping from the shower. As I run across the street, I can hear the turbine winding up on the helicopter on the roof. The day crew member is holding the door open for me as well as holding out the radio and keys, which I grab on the fly.

Jogging through the ED, I do see Drena sitting at the nurse's table in the hallway, and she smiles and laughs when she sees me in my current wardrobe. I smile and wave as I pass by and arrive at the elevator to find the security guard there, holding it for me. I step in, thanking him, and put the key into the slot that will give me an express ride up to the roof. As I ride up, I finish zipping up my boots and pull up my flight suit. By the time the doors open on the roof, I have my helmet on and start running up the ramp to the running ship. As I round the corner, I can see that Bruce is already in and has left the sliding door open for me so I can just jump in. After snapping my seat belt, I give Marty a thumbs-up and he lifts the ship off the rooftop as I continue to fasten my flight bag under the seat and finally plug my helmet into the intercom. As I do this, Bruce, looking at me, smiling, welcomes me with a "Glad you could make it. Can we go now?"

I just smile and thank them for waiting, then ask where we are going. Marty answers that we are going up around the Downieville area for someone that fell off a horse. I look up at them, and now thinking they are screwing with me, I ask, "Really, is that what we are going for?"

"Yes," answers Bruce. Then he adds, "Why do you ask?"

I then tell them, "That was the reason I was almost late. I was out for a ride on Joe. Go figure!"

We laugh, and as we put in the coordinates and look it up on the map, I know where we are going. It is near the area I grew up. I then tell them that this area is really steep and the mountains are granite and volcanic with very jagged peaks, but hopefully, there is a place to land close to the patient.

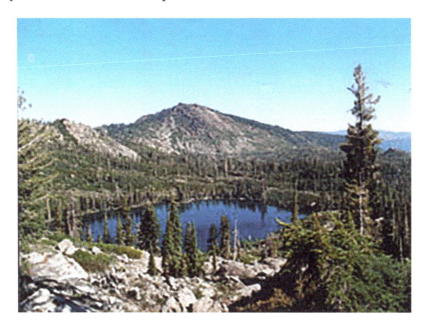

As we near the area, we give the Downieville Fire Department a call on the radio, and they quickly answer. They fill us in that the coordinates they have given us is only the spot where they are and that they not only haven't made it to the patient yet but are only guessing she is about a mile or two from them. This information has been relayed to them from another rider that has ridden out to call for help. They then tell us that there are still several other riders still with the woman and to look for several horses. We acknowledge this, and as we pass over the ridge of the mountain, we can see the lakes of Gold Lake Basin, and it is simply beautiful.

HORSING AROUND

As we pass over the ridge, I look down and can see the group of fire vehicles and an ambulance. Marty starts dropping some altitude, and I open the sliding door and turn in my seat so I can get a better view out the door, looking down for any signs of people, horses, or anyone. It doesn't take long before I look out and can see a half-dozen horses tied up to some trees and just as many people waving frantically at us. "There they are!" I tell Bruce as Marty starts banking the ship over to get closer to them.

As we start into a couple recon circles over the riders, I see one person lying on the ground and tell the crew, "Yes, this is it. That must be our patient." Then as we continue to circle, looking for a suitable landing spot, it becomes very apparent that there isn't one. We fly out some distance, broadening our circles, and still come up with the same answer: there is nowhere to land.

Plan B. We decide to contact the fire department and see if they have anyone starting into the scene yet, and they tell us that their four-wheel-drive ambulance has made it about a mile in but could go no farther but three of the personnel are hiking in. They have seen where we are circling the scene and now know where to go. They fill us in that they will be bringing in a backboard and some equipment but it is going to take them anywhere from thirty to forty-five minutes to reach the patient and they are just basic life support.

Bruce and I look at each other and now know what we will have to do. One of us will have to be dropped off and start caring for the patient and await for the fire department rescuers to arrive to assist in hauling the patient out. Marty and I are now looking for a suitable location that he can get close enough to the ground that we can either do a one-skid landing or hover close enough that I can jump out, then Bruce will drop the first-out bag to me. We finally decide on a location that we can get close enough to the ground that Marty can hover, which in itself will be challenging, as we are well over seven thousand feet in elevation.

As I prepare myself, I watch as Marty slows the ship and lets it drop down until we are about five feet above the ground, and looking at the brush below us, I tell him to stop and that we cannot descend any further. He tells me that he is okay holding the elevation, and I quickly release my seat belt and pull my helmet off, handing it to

Bruce. I turn as I step out onto the step on the skid, then step down to the lower skid, holding on to the doors of the helicopter, looking down, trying to decide if I want to try to step off or just jump. I finally see the spot I think is the best, and with a slight turn and releasing my grip on the doors, I step off into the air.

What I think is going to be about a five-foot drop really ends up to be about eight by the time my legs settle down through some of the brush. I drop to my knees as my feet tangle themselves, dropping into the brush, and when my hands finally contact the ground, I know I'm not hurt and, in all aspects, have made a successful landing. I straighten myself up in the brush, then decide to step over to a very small opening, where I will have better footing, and after doing so, I look up at Bruce and motion for him to toss me the bag.

When you are standing below a hovering helicopter and someone is looking out down at you then drops something at you, it looks a whole lot bigger than it really is, and because I have done this several times, I know that you don't want to try to catch it. The fairly heavy bag loaded with medical gear and IV solutions gains speed in the drop and can knock you over. What I have learned is to just raise my hands, and when it makes contact, just slow its descent and let it fall to the ground or try to steer it to a bush for a softer landing, and this is exactly what I do. I feel the bag slapping my hands, which are over my head, and I quickly push them in front of me, letting the bag come to rest in a bush, breaking its fall. Looking up, I give Bruce a thumbs-up, and the two of them turn and start flying off toward the ridgeline. Then after pulling out the shoulder straps and attaching them to the bag, I strap it onto my back and start hiking to where I believe the patient is.

After hiking about a half-mile, I am met by a person that I am guessing is from the group. She is wearing a cowboy hat, boots, and spurs. Not your everyday mountain hiker.

"Boy, are we glad to see you!" she says with some excitement in her voice. "We thought we might have to spend the night up here."

"Well, don't get too excited yet," I tell her. "We still need to figure out how we are going to get her out of here."

As we continue walking to where the rest of the party is, she starts telling me about the injured woman. That they are a group of women who ride together often and were all out riding the summit trail on this beautiful day and, for unknown reasons, the injured woman's horse made a quick move and the woman lost her balance and simply fell off. At first, all the remaining girls laughed, as it looked fairly harmless and, in reality, looked as if she went to the ground slowly and no one dreamed she would be hurt. But when the woman tried to get up, she could feel pain running down her leg and couldn't move. I then ask if she knows anything else about her, if she has any medical problems, or maybe her age, and the woman fills me in on what she knows.

After about a fifteen-minute hike, talking with the woman, I start to hear the horses, and as we emerge from the timber, I am met with a group of cowgirls. I am then greeted with everything from very worried people to laughing that they still can't believe she's hurt herself. As I work my way through the women, who all seem to want to talk to me, I finally reach my patient lying on the ground and introduce myself. "I'm Greg. What's your name?"

As she looks up at me, I can see worry in her face as she answers, "Samantha, I'm Samantha, but everyone calls me Sam."

"Okay, Sam, tell me what you remember about what happened here and where you are hurting."

As she starts with her story, I start examining her, and when I finally push on her hips, she lets out a very stern grimace. I continue to check down her legs, and even though she does not want to move her left leg, she can still feel me touching her leg and foot. I decide to remove her boots, and sure enough, I find what I have been afraid of—her left foot is slightly shorter than the right and rotated out to the side. As I study this, she picks up on the fact that I have found something and asks, "So, Doc, what do you think?"

Smiling, I start filling her in on what I know. "Well, Sam, first of all, I'm not a doctor, I'm a nurse. Second of all, I believe you have fractured your left hip."

"Are you shitting me?"

"No, that is what it is looking like, but you really need an x-ray to confirm that. But I guarantee you"—now I point to her left hip—"something is broken in there." I then decide to fill her in on what to expect next. "So here is our plan. I'm going to start an IV on you, and I can give you some morphine to help with the pain. Then we will be waiting for the fire department personnel to hike into here so we can put you on a spinal board and carry you out."

"That doesn't sound like much fun," she says as I am pulling the IV equipment out of the bag.

I then tell her that I really have no idea how far we will have to carry her, but the fire department personnel will fill us in on that when they arrive, and because I haven't seen where the helicopter has finally landed after dropping me off, they may be anywhere but probably on top of the hill, and it may be quite a hike.

As I'm starting the IV and pushing some morphine, I ask her about her horse and tell her that I have just been riding mine an hour ago. At the same time, I can't help but think that there must be a way I can convince the fire department guys and gals to carry her out and I'll ride her horse out. As I mention this in my conversation to her, she tells me that that would be great if I would. I then tell her that I'll try to work it out.

About twenty minutes after arriving at the cowgirls, I hear one of the ladies saying, "Here come the firefighters." I stand up and look to where she is pointing and see three men pushing themselves through some brush, following a vague trail. As they arrive, they set the board down, and it is quite obvious that these guys are worn-out from the hike, and what worries me is that part of the hike has been downhill.

I recognize the captain, as I have taught many classes in Downieville, and ask him what the plan is. He then starts telling me that we are going to have to carry the patient for about two miles. The first mile is fairly flat, but we have to walk around the lake's edge until we reach a trail that goes up the hill. He then starts telling us that the so-called trail up the hill is over large boulders and is almost straight up. I then ask if there is any good news in the conversation, and he tells me, "Yes, the ambulance is going to be able to drive about halfway down the hill and will meet us there."

Now, as he points to some fictitious place on the hill, and not seeing anything that looks like an ambulance, I just nod.

"Well, let's get her loaded up and get to this," I say to everyone.

The firefighters help in placing Sam onto the board and securing her. I give her another dose of morphine and tell her that I'll keep this in my pocket and for her to tell me if she needs any more. Then looking up and seeing Sam's horse, I tell her that it doesn't sound like I'm going to be able to ride him out. The firefighters agree, telling us that there is no way a horse is going to be able to go where we will be going, which doesn't help our attitude. One of the other ladies then speaks up and tells Sam that she will pony her horse back with her and take care of him. Sam thanks her, and with that, I motion for the fire personnel to lift the board.

After throwing my first-out bag onto my back, I grab one of the corners, and the four of us start out. At first, the trail that works its way to the lake is fairly simple, and I start to think to myself, *This isn't too bad.* Once we are at the lake, we start around the shoreline, and as we are walking, the captain starts telling us that the trail ends soon and we will be wading through the water to get around a rockslide. He has no sooner said this than I see the slide, and the two firefighters in the front start into the water. Before we are ten or fifteen feet from the shoreline, it is already up to our waist, and we are starting to have to hold Sam up high enough to keep her out of the water. "How deep is this going to get?" I ask, not sure I really want an answer but hope it doesn't mean we will be swimming.

"About a foot deeper," one of the firefighters says as he turns and now starts to push the board up to about the height of his neck.

At this point, all I can think of is, *Shit, I didn't have a chance to get all my books and papers out of my lower-leg pockets.* Then a second thought goes through me as I suddenly remember, *My radio! My boss is going to kill me!*

I am now holding my corner of the board up to my neck, and the water is about midchest, and the four of us are having trouble finding footing. A couple of times, we have almost lost the board as one of us stumbles as we slowly try to walk by braille, not seeing where we are placing our feet. As we slowly make our way around the end of the rockslide, I suddenly hear a different voice and look up to see that there are a couple more firefighters standing on the shoreline. They have hiked down from the ambulance and decided to wait at the water's edge, as they didn't know where the other had gone. They step into the water, and now with the six of us each helping steady the board with Sam on it, we make faster progress and, within moments, are out of the water and on the shoreline. I then ask the group to set her down so I can make sure things are okay, and in reality, we need a break.

As I bend over to talk to Sam, I ask, "How are you doing?"

She looks me directly in the eyes and says, "That was about the scariest damn thing I have ever had to do in my life. I thought you guys were going to drop me a couple of times, and being tied to this board, I just knew I was going to flip upside down and drown."

I let out a smile and tell her, "I agree, and in reality, it was pretty damn scary from our side also." I then give her another dose of morphine, which I know will help settle her nerves, and since I have no idea what the next part of our journey is, I decide it may be a bumpy haul up the hill.

After placing the syringe back into my pocket, I ask one of the new fire personnel how much farther it is, and looking up the hill, he tells us, "It isn't really that far, maybe half a mile, but—"

I cut him off and finish his sentence, "It's all uphill!"

Looking at me with a smile, he nods. "Yup, you got it."

I take a deep breath and tell the others, "Okay, let's get this done."

We take our places and, now with the two extra firefighters, start up the incredibly steep hill. Several times, different people slip and we all concentrate on making sure that Sam isn't dropped. A couple of times, we have had to set the board down on a boulder and have two of us push it up while the rest pull it up and over the top of a boulder. After about twenty minutes of doing this, we have found that what works best while we are hiking up the hill is to have four people carrying the board, one on each corner, and the remaining two in the rear, pushing the two on the rear of the board. Not only is the added push helpful, but this also seems to stabilize us as we are not slipping or stumbling nearly as bad as when the four of us have started out.

We finally push through one last large patch of manzanita, and right in front of us is the ambulance. The gurney is already out, and we walk alongside it and gently set Sam down. "We made it," I tell her, but looking down at her, I can tell the ride up the hill has not been fun for her; at times, she has nearly been vertical, and the weight of her body has been putting pressure on her fractured hip. "Not much farther now," I tell her, but in reality, looking up the so-called road, I know this is going to be a very rough ride in the four-wheel-drive ambulance.

As we all climb into the back of the Chevy Suburban, I can't help but ask one of the Downieville firefighters, "Isn't this the old Sierraville ambulance?"

"Yes. How do you know that?" he asks.

I then tell him that this very ambulance was where I started my career in emergency services. As I look around inside, I can see they have made a few modifications, and as we start out up the hill, I can feel the four-wheel-drive biting into the dirt and rocks. At times we are tossed almost violently around in the back, with the driver shouting, "Sorry!" each time. I know he is doing his best and is trying to make this trip as smooth as possible, but in reality, even though he is only doing about one-half a mile per hour, it isn't.

I dose Sam with the last of the morphine after taking her vital signs, then, looking out the window, ask the driver, "How much farther to the helicopter?" I have no idea where it is, and as far as I know, it may be all the way down the other side of the hill in town.

"Not much farther. They were able to land somewhere up there," he says, pointing out the front window, but not really at anything, as he can't hold his arm straight enough as he is being tossed around just as much as we are.

I have my arms out to the sides, not only to hold myself in one place, but also to try to keep Sam from moving too much. Two of the firefighters have chosen to not ride in the ambulance but to hike up the hill, and one of them has passed us and is now leading the rig up the hill. We are being tossed around so much that I am now thinking seriously that it may be better for Sam if we take her out of the ambulance and carry her up the hill, and just as I lean forward, looking out the windshield of the ambulance to tell the driver that maybe we should consider walking, I see something sticking out of the brush ahead of us. After a couple more bumps, I make out the tail boom of the helicopter.

I take a second look to make sure that is what I am seeing, and sure enough, I can make out the blue, silver, and red stripes. We are still in a very thick, forested area, and I am totally shocked that Marty was able to land here. As we pull up alongside the helicopter, I can make out the crew and a couple other firefighters and sheriff officers. As we come to a stop, I tell Sam that we have finally made it, that we will have her out of here and into the helicopter in just a few moments, and promise her a nice, smooth ride to Chico. As we pull her from the back of the ambulance and move her over to the flight gurney, she grabs my hand and tells me to please thank the others for getting her out. "You can do that yourself," I tell her, and as she opens her eyes, she can now see almost all the crew that has helped her in her ordeal.

"Thank you all from the bottom of my heart!" she says, followed by most of the crew walking up and either shaking her hand or patting her on her shoulders.

We slide her into the ship, and after attaching some equipment and pulling out another morphine vial, I administer some of the medication to her for the flight to Chico. Marty starts up the ship and pulls us straight up and out of the forest, and as he makes his turn to the west and home, I can see the sun setting in the distance.

"We weren't sure you were going to get out of there in time," Marty tells me, then asks, "How was the hike?"

I personally think he is joking, as I am covered in dirt and mud, my arms are covered in scratches from the thick manzanita, and my boots are full of water. Then remembering my equipment, I pull the radio off my waist, and as I open the battery, the three of us watch as water pours out. "Oh, man, the boss is going to kick your ass!" Bruce says with a big smile on his face, followed by Marty asking, "How many radios is that for you, four or five, right?"

Trying to shake some more water out of the unit, I count and say, "I think this is number six, but who's counting?"

We all start laughing, and knowing this radio is now toast, I just toss the pieces down onto the floor.

After we have landed and unloaded Sam in the orthopedic room, Bruce has agreed to gather equipment and put the ship together while I go attempt to clean up a little. I walk into the nurse's lounge and pull off my boots, emptying the remaining water into the sink, then remove my socks, wring them out, and hang them over the back of a chair. I then start pulling out of my pockets my books and papers, which I keep with different aids to anything from IV medication drips, burn charts, and phone numbers. They are all soaked, and as I am trying to pull them apart, I hear the door open and look up to see Drena walk in. She takes one look at my muddy suit, scratched arms and face, wet socks hanging on the chair and starts laughing. "Can't wait to hear this story," she says, placing a hand on my shoulder.

"Help me try to save my papers," I ask, handing her one of my books.

The two of us continue to try to open the different pages that are stuck together and dry them off or place them out on a towel on the table to dry as I tell her about my mountain exploit.

I ask her if she's had a chance to talk to Sam yet, and she tells me she has and she's gotten enough information from her to contact some of her family members. A sister is now en route here, and a brother will go to her house and help out when her horse arrives. She then remembers something she's told her and asks, "Hey, do you know what the name of the lake is that you were at?"

I think for a moment, knowing most of the lakes in that area, but finally admit that I don't know that one. "No, what was it?"

"That was Horse Lake," she tells me.

I look at her, stunned. "Are you kidding me?" I ask, not really wanting an answer, then tell her, "This must be the day of the horse. I rode my horse today, went to a woman who fell from a horse, and of all things, went wading in Horse Lake. Unbelievable!"

We laugh, then she adds, "Aren't you glad it isn't the day of the pig?"

16

IDLE TIME

Paul

AS YOU HAVE probably learned by now, there are three essential parts of the emergency medical services (EMS): One, being good at your job. Two, handling very stressful situations. And three, screwing around during downtime. It seems that everyone involved in EMS likes to joke around. This is a big part of this work and helps keep the day-to-day stress at bay. If you are the type that doesn't like anyone pulling jokes, especially on you, then you should consider a career change, because if the others figure out that you don't like to be joked with, you will instantly become their primary focus during any of their downtime.

For a very long time, every shift I would take in Oroville, my boss, Paul, would try to pull something on me. In reality, he didn't have much of a sense of humor and most of the staff couldn't figure out what he was trying to do, and after his failed attempt at humor, he would just laugh out loud, mainly to himself, as he thought he had pulled off some incredible prank. The rest of us would only laugh because we knew he really hadn't accomplished anything, but he was our boss, so going along with his laughter was the right thing to do.

Oroville ran three ambulances, two of which were the first-out rigs, one stationed in the west side of the district, in a cockroach-infested suburb known as Thermalito. The other was stationed at the hospital in the east side of the district. Both of these were staffed with a crew of three, two paramedics and one EMT. The third ambulance was the transfer rig. It was responsible for, you got it, all the transfers. The transfer rig was only staffed with two, an EMT and a paramedic. The paramedic staffed on this rig was also the charge paramedic for the shift and responsible for anything that might come up during the day and needed some type of administrative decision, mainly sick calls. You were also the backup rig if the other two rigs were busy or out of position.

I remember one such shift when I was assigned to the transfer unit. The other two first-out rigs were each sent to calls at the farthest point of our coverage area, which would keep them gone for one to two hours at a time, and they were canceled each time. My EMT partner and I had to cover the entire Oroville area by ourselves. By the time our shift had ended, both of the first-out rigs had run a total of eight calls; the two of us on the transfer rig had run twenty-six, which included two transfers to Chico and one to Sacramento.

One day, I had been called at my job at Enloe by the charge paramedic in Oroville, and he asked if I could come over and cover a shift the next day. He had not one but two different sick calls; the first was for a first-out rig, which our boss, Paul, said he would cover. The second one that came in was for the charge paramedic on the transfer rig. "Sure," I told him. I could use the extra money, as I was buying my new truck. I also thought in the back of my head that as Paul was scheduled, he would switch with me and take the charge spot. This would also keep him at the hospital, and he could walk out to his office to catch up on some paperwork or work on his sense of humor.

By the time I got to the quarters the next morning, I had decided to give him a hard time and play with his ego a little. He had been trying to pull something over on me for years, and I decided this was my chance to pull one on him. When I walked into the quarters, one of the first-out rigs from yesterday was just arriving, and walking into the office to report off, as the four of us walked in, I looked up at the board and my name was still listed as the charge paramedic. The rest of the new crews were coming in, and I decided to go ahead and start briefing them on what little I knew when Paul walked in. I didn't even slow down with my report, and when he attempted to change the names on the assignment board, I stopped him, asking, "What do you think you are doing?"

Stunned, he looked at me for a moment, then started to say, "Well, I thought I'd take the charge spot and you coul—"

I cut him off by saying, "You thought wrong. Now, let me finish my report."

I knew it was a brave thing to do, and I could see several of the EMTs and paramedics snickering; after all, this was just a part-time job for me. The worst thing that could happen was I just wouldn't be called back for any shifts.

Paul stepped away from the board, and after I finished my report, the offgoing crews filled in the new crews if anything needed to be done to the rigs and handed off the keys and radios. I had already met with the offgoing charge paramedic and had my keys and radio, keeping Paul from grabbing them. As the old crews were gathering their bags and bedrolls and heading home, the new crews were doing the same, and everyone was walking out to find their rigs to start checking them. Standing outside of mine, Paul walked up and asked me again if I wanted to take the first-out rig, and now knowing I had to stick to my guns, I gave him a polite, "No, I'm good. Thanks for asking."

Throughout the remainder of the day, he asked about trading several times, but I decided that wasn't going to happen. I liked Diana, the EMT I was working with, and we were already having a great day. Paul, on the other hand, was assigned with two women who were great at their jobs but had decided to give him a hard time all day long. Each time I would see them as they brought in a patient, the girls would smile and say they were having a great time.

By the time darkness had fallen, my partner and I were trying to come up with something to do to Paul that would really get his goat. It was around eleven o'clock in the evening when we hear Paul's rig get dispatched down Highway 70 to the most southern part of our area. "Jump in, let's go!" I shouted to Diana.

"Where are we going?" she asked as we ran to our rig.

"Thermalito" was all I had to say.

She didn't exactly know what I had in mind, but the only thing out there was the small house the hospital had rented for the west-side crew to stay in. As we drove through town, she asked questions on what we were going to do, and all I could say was, "I'm not sure yet. We need to get there, look around, and I'm sure some inspiration will strike us." Smiling, the two of us raced out to the west side and pulled up to the small house. We all had keys, so entering wasn't a problem. The thing about Thermalito was, the town was a dump. No one would be out after dark, the bugs were incredible, as the town followed the Feather River, and we always locked ourselves into the building.

As we walked through the house, I was trying to come up with something to do when I looked into one of the bedrooms. "I've got it!" I told Diana. The house had two bedrooms; one had one bed in it, while the other room had two beds in it. This way, if you had a crew of two women and one man, or the opposite, it worked out. I knew the two girls would be staying in the room with the two beds, and Paul would be staying in the room with the one bed. As I flipped on the light, I could see a duffel bag and instantly knew this was Paul's stuff.

As Diana came in, I filled her in on my diabolical plan. "Let's take everything out of the bedroom and put it all in the backyard."

"Cool!" she said, and without further discussion, we started hauling everything outside, table lamp, table, phone, Paul's bag, and Paul's bed. We then took a moment to set up everything out in the yard just as it appeared in the room. Make the bed, set up the table, phone, and lamp at the bedside, and set Paul's bag on the bed just as we found it. Then, the two of us stood back to admire our work, smiling and laughing when we heard Paul's rig call in that the patient had signed AMA and they would be returning to quarters.

"Shit!" both of us said as we ran through the house, shutting off all the lights and dashing out to our rig. We knew we had to get back to town and under the freeway overpass before they returned and saw us in their area, which might throw off the joke. Diana hauled ass across the surface streets, crossed the bridge, and as we went under the freeway, I looked to see if I could see the other rig and, not seeing them, started laughing, knowing our plan was in motion.

The remainder of the evening went fairly normal, and we didn't have any further contact with the other two crews. By morning, I had almost forgotten about the prank as I was filling in the oncoming charge paramedic on a few things when Paul and his crew came into the office. The two girls were laughing and walking up to the two of us, saying, "That was so cool! You have no idea how funny that was!" The new crews were puzzled and started asking what happened, and Paul was trying to change the subject, but the two girls that were with him wouldn't let it lie. They started in by telling the new three crews and the other crew from our shift about it. That they had been out on several calls, and finally, around one in the morning, they were crashed on the sofas, watching TV, when Paul decided to go to bed. He got up and walked to his room and flipped on the light switch and nothing happened. Now, flipping it up and down several times, he said, "What is going on?" The girls just sat on the sofa, watching him, and one of them told him that she thought they didn't have any replacement light bulbs and he would have to use his flashlight. He then entered his room to retrieve his light from his bag and found nothing. Now louder, he yelled at the girls and they came to the room. One of them shone her light in, and all that was in the room was Paul. The two of them started laughing, especially when Paul became concerned about his bag and bedroll. The three of them then started looking around, and after about five minutes, one of them looked out into the backyard and, turning on the rear porch light, found the entire bedroom set. The two girls burst out laughing, and as Paul walked out to see his new room, he told them, "This isn't funny. I'm not sleeping out here!" The two girls, still laughing, filled him in that their bedroom was okay and they felt no obligation to help him move back in. As a matter of fact, the two of them sat on the sofa and watched as he dragged everything back into the house and set it up back in his room.

All the crews were now laughing, and Paul was shaking his head, knowing he was the butt of the joke, and I also knew he would make it his destiny to get back at me.

IDLE TIME

As the crews started out of the office, on their way home or to their rigs, several of them slapped me on the back with a "Well done!"

As I finished with what I had to do and gathered my gear, I walked up to Paul and, sticking out my hand, asked, "No hard feelings?"

He took my hand and, not letting go, squeezed hard and finally said, "No, no hard feelings. You got me."

We chatted for a while, and before walking out the door, he added one last thing, that he would get his revenge. I smiled and, as the door was closing, told him, "Good luck!"

The Phone Drill (Sorry, Mike)

"You know, Mike has been here on night shift for over a month, and he seems to be developing an attitude," Pam tells me.

"You know, I think you're right." I pause, thinking the situation over and also thinking about the pleas from my boss: "Do not scare him off! We like him and want him to stay here. Understand?" I know the night shift can be hard on new employees, but we also feel that they need a full, undisrupted orientation to exactly how things are done on the night shift. As a matter of fact, our motto is, "What are they going to do, put us on nights?" We know we do a few things a little differently than day shift, usually a little more efficiently; we also know we like the fact that we don't have all the administration walking through, checking up on us day after day, week after week, and finally, know that our boss will overlook some of the hazing and jokes as long as we continue to show up for our shifts and she doesn't have to worry about filling vacant night shifts.

Mike had worked at Enloe years ago as an EMT, putting himself through nursing school, and when he finished, he moved his family to Hawaii and started his nursing career, working in one of the island hospitals. After several years, island fever had set in and they had decided to move back to the mainland. Both he and his wife had been raised in the Chico area, so upon returning, he had reapplied to work at Enloe. Now working in the same hospital but now as a nurse, he seems to think he is immune to any pranking, and he couldn't be more wrong.

"You know, you're right. It may be time to put him in his place and give him a big 'Welcome to night shift!'" I say with a smile, totally dismissing the boss's disclaimer about being nice to the new guy. Pam and I then put our minds together, trying to pick which of the normal welcomes we should bestow on him when our night dispatcher speaks up.

"You know, I have asked Mike several times to come into dispatch and get oriented, and each time he has refused, saying, 'I don't need to do that. I'll never be in there except to take a radio report.'"

Pam and I then look at each other and simultaneously say, "Phone drill!"

The phone drill is usually quick and easy. The dispatcher will ask someone to cover them so they can go to lunch or the bathroom, and as soon as they leave, we place a bogus call into dispatch then watch and listen as the panic sets in on our prey. In Mike's case, we decide that we need to take this maybe a little further than normal, since Mike has EMT experience and there is a possibility that he will catch on.

Before we know it, we have the entire department in on it. It seems that everyone wants to put the fear of God into Mike. Everyone plans a different scenario to call in with, and we hand out the different phone numbers that should be used. As an added measure, we also call the 911 dispatcher to let them in on the gag, knowing that Mike might call them, requesting aid from another ambulance or fire department to be dispatched. They must be just as bored as we are, as they buy right into it and say they will play into it until we call and tell them it is over.

Now with everyone set in their roles, we all sit at the nurse's station, looking as if we are actually doing something, and wait for our prey. Soon, we see Mike walking up the hallway, carrying a newspaper, and just as he is passing the entrance to dispatch, the dispatcher steps out and, without stopping, says to Mike, "Hey, buddy, would you mind watching the phone for a minute while I run to the men's room? Thanks!" He then slaps him on the shoulder and turns away before Mike can try to talk himself out of the request. The dispatcher continues to walk down the hall as Mike takes a look at all the nursing staff sitting at the nursing station, not looking at him, but concentrating on different charts, paperwork, talking on phones, all looking really busy. He finally shrugs his shoulders and turns into dispatch, sits in the chair right in front of the large console, and opens his paper.

I slowly look up over the counter, and when I see him becoming very comfortable and putting his feet up on another chair, I give the signal for the rest of the staff to commence. We all jump from our seats but stay crouched over so he cannot see us leaving, then run out of the department to different phones in different room. In fact, we totally abandon the nurse's station; this way, if he looks out for help, there won't be any.

Mike has now become overly comfortable in the dispatch chair, not paying any attention to the console, which has twenty different emergency lines programmed into it. Most of which have red buttons that will flash when a call comes in. There are also three FlightCare lines with the same red buttons, but a different ringtone. Add to this different white lines that are regular phone lines, and don't forget the TTY phone, which is for the person at home that is deaf and mute. There are also three radios. Two are dispatch radios, and one is the medical radio for taking radio reports from the field. Not a place to park your overconfident self, especially on a slow night shift.

Mike jumps from his seat when the first loud ring goes off, and when he looks down, he can see one of the red lines flashing. He picks up the phone receiver and pushes the flashing button, answering, "Uh, this is Enloe dispatch, what's your emergency?" As he is now searching for something to write on and write with—which he will not find, as the dispatcher has hidden all the writing tools—the caller on the other end starts telling him how she is in labor and thinks she needs an ambulance, then tells him to hang on for a minute as another contraction is about to start, then she starts screaming into the phone. At this time, a second ring starts filling the room, and Mike looks down and sees another red line lighting up.

ON THE GO

As it continues to blare and flash, he yells back at the woman in labor, telling her that he has to put her on hold for a moment. He pushes the Hold button, then answers the second flashing light and finds a hysterical male voice yelling at him, "There is an accident on the highway, and there are several people lying on the road, all bleeding and all needing an ambulance!" Mike is now breaking into a sweat, and not finding anything to write on, he pulls the pen out of his pocket and is now writing on the palm of his hand and trying to put notes down when a third, different ring fills the room. Cutting the man off midsentence, telling him to hold for a moment, he pushes the Hold button and now sees one of the FlightCare lines flashing. He answers the call. "Enloe FlightCare, how can I help you?"

"This is Dr. Mindless calling from Quincy. I have a very unstable cardiac patient that needs to be flown to Chico."

Now knowing that things are totally out of control, he pulls the phone as far as it will reach out of dispatch, yelling for someone to come help him, but when he looks out to the nurse's station, there is no one there. *No one!*

Walking back to the console and now not sitting but standing, as if that will help, he tells the physician to hang on for a moment and pushes the Hold button. Now totally panicked, he decides to reach out to the county 911 system and attempt to get help. He pushes the red line with the 911 on it, and one of the county dispatchers answers, "Nine-one-one, please hold!" and with a click, he places him on hold. Mike holds the phone out in front of him and stares at it in disbelief, then looking back at the console, which is now flashing multiple colors and patterns of new calls and holding calls, he pushes the first button and hears the pregnant woman still screaming. He places it back on hold and pushes the second button, and the man on the highway starts yelling at him, "Where the hell did you go? One of these dudes looks really bad! He is now having a seizure and is flopping all over the highway!"

"Shit!" Mike says, looking out to the nurse's station once again for help when he pushes one of the new red lines and is met with the multiple tones of the TTY phone sending a coded message to the digital receiver in dispatch. But not knowing or just not caring at this point, he just hangs up and answers the FlightCare line. "Dr. Mindless, are you still there?" he asks with a quiver in his voice.

"What the hell? Are you going to come get this guy, or do I need to call another helicopter?"

"No, don't do that. We will be up there as soon as we can." Then with close to ten lines flashing, he tells him once again, "Please hold."

About then, Pam walks into the room and can see Mike holding two phones and dripping sweat like he is in the shower and asks, "What the hell are you doing?"

Mike looks up at her with a total look of someone lost and, pointing to the flashing lines, starts in, "There's some woman having a baby." He points to another. "There is an accident on the highway." Then he points to the FlightCare line and says, "And Dr. Mindless in Quincy needs the helicopter."

Pam, somehow keeping a straight face, then tells him, "You have to page the flight crew!"

Mike now knows he can't even answer all the calls and, having no idea how to set off the pagers, asks her, "Can you page out the crew?"

Pam then tells him that she doesn't know how to do it but continues to tell him that he must push the paging buttons, and after Mike tells her that he doesn't know how to do that, she tells him that maybe he can just mimic the tones. "If you push the transmit button on the radio and make the proper tones, it might set off the pagers." Mike, still holding two phones, one of which is the screaming pregnant woman, just looks at her in total disbelief when Pam continues, "Yes, I think you can do that. I believe the tones sound something like…" She then goes into what is an imitation of the three different tones. "UH-UHHHH, then UHHHH-OOOOO, and I believe the third one sounds something like BLAHHHH-BAAAAHH!"

Mike is now buried, knowing he can't do that, but in the back of his mind, he thinks, *I may have to try.* When he turns from Pam and back to the console, trying to answer another call, Pam starts to leave the room. He then turns to her, yelling, "Go find that dispatcher and tell him to get back up here!" Mike then tries to call the 911 dispatcher back and, once again, is taken aback when he is told,

"Please hold." As he is now deciding he has two choices, to try to talk all these people through their tragedies or just simply drop the phones on the desk and run from the building and go look for a job flipping burgers at McDonald's, he then looks up to see all of us have walked into dispatch and are laughing so hard we are having trouble standing.

Mike just stands there, looking at us, two phones tangled together, not knowing why we aren't helping him and, at the same time, pushing different buttons and finding that no one is on the other end of the phone lines anymore. Then it suddenly hits him, and he just stands there, letting his arms drop to his side, sweat running from his face, and watches as all the once flashing, beeping, and buzzing lines go out one by one then all become silent. Now knowing he has been had, he lets out with a, "Shit!" as he places the phones back onto the receivers. "That wasn't funny!" he tries to tell us, but we are all laughing so hard all of us have tears in our eyes. The girls are having trouble not wetting their panties, and I'm totally bent over, holding my stomach.

Mike decides to take a stroll down the hall and out onto the ambulance dock to let the night air cool him off a little as we call the 911 dispatchers, who now want to hear the entire story, and after filling them in, we thank them for once again helping us. I can only hope that Mike is a good enough sport and can take the joke, and after a few minutes, he strolls back into the ED and it is very apparent that he can, as he then thanks us all for initiating him into the night shift world, shaking our hands and giving us a slap on the back. Before he finishes thanking the last coworker, he is already thinking up some redemption and asks, "Whom can we get next?"

I worked with Mike as my primary partner on and off over the next ten-plus years, and I must say, we worked incredibly well as a team and had become very good friends. He's never forgotten the phone drill we pulled on him that night and was always a part of doing the same to other new staff members over the years.

Dr. Bowman's Memorial AIDS Package

I remember in my EMT class in 1983, our teacher, who had been an ER nurse in the surrounding communities for many years, was well respected, and if you passed her class, that was saying something. At the end of the class, we were all stressed out about the final exam, and I just about choked up when one of the last essay questions read, "What does *AAA* stand for?" I skipped the question and came back to it, thinking the answer would pop into my head. By the time I was reviewing my exam, I was down to that one last question, thinking, *What in the EMS world would* AAA *stand for?* Finally, with myself and only one more student still in the room, I filled in the answer, "American Automobile Association," and turned it in.

Leaving the classroom, I found all the students were outside, discussing the test, all stressed out on what everyone had answered to all the different questions. I finally asked, "Does anyone know what triple A stands for?" I guess 80 percent of the class had put the same answer as I did, the American Automobile Association. The best we could come up with why they would ask such a question was that maybe you should know who the insurance company might be when you were on a motor-vehicular accident. After the last student left the classroom, we cornered our instructor on her way out, and we had to ask her what the answer was. When we told her our answer was the insurance company, she laughed, then told us that that wasn't the answer but, in fact, she couldn't remember the correct answer either.

Something I have disagreed with throughout my career is, when you take a test, you get the results, a grade, but you don't get the correct answers to the questions you may have missed. Most of the time, you really won't know what you missed. You get a 90 percent, smile, and go through life thinking your answers must have been okay. In reality, you may go years or an entire career not knowing the correct answer to a question, and does that mean you are mistreating a patient, thinking your answer was correct? It wasn't until my first recert class in Butte College that I learned that AAA stood for "ascending aortic aneurysm."

Such was the case with another set of abbreviations, AIDS. When I started as an EMT, AIDS was the name of an ambulance service in Reno, Nevada. At that time, those letters stood for the name of the people who owned the company; it wasn't for another five years that those four letters would represent one of the scariest diseases known to mankind. Once that happened, no one wanted to be transported in an ambulance with the big four letters on the doors. Why not have an ambulance called typhoid transport, smallpox ambulance, or syphilis EMS? At that time, I remember the joke of the day was, "Why is Reno the only city with a gay rodeo?" The answer being, "Because they're the only city with an AIDS ambulance." As you can guess, by the mideighties, that company was doomed.

It wasn't until I was in paramedic school when we were really introduced to what AIDS really was and how it was affecting the nation and the world. Being in California, it was a real threat to EMS workers, and we really didn't know how we would react when our first contact would be made. We were all very well educated on the disease but still scared to death of it.

I remember, when the first contact was made in Chico, the paramedic was so scared that it took her four attempts to start an IV. Each time looking at the now-contaminated needle and watching as blood was running from the start sites. We would eventually come to know and treat the AIDS patients as no other than any of our normal, everyday patients, and in reality, that was all they were. But that didn't mean we couldn't have a little fun with the national scare at that time.

Once again, it's night shift. It's around two in the morning on a Wednesday, and we have no patients in the ED. *None!* What does that mean? It means it is time to pull something off on someone. Mike and I have been walking around, looking for something to do, which in itself usually leads to getting into trouble when we decide that our new EMT, Mark, working in dispatch, needs to be welcomed into the night shift family. He has been working here for about a week, and we can tell he is feeling a little overconfident with himself. He's had some EMS experience somewhere in the past and has been orienting to the ambulance and to dispatch. Tonight, he is the dispatcher. Looking into the small room just off the ED, we know we need to do something. *Phone drill?* No. Did that last week. How about the dead-guy-in-the-ambulance trick? No, we think he has heard of that one when the day shift told him he was going to nights and gave him a list of things to watch out for. No, we are going to have to come up with something totally new. Now our diabolical minds really start in. First of all, we know what we want to accomplish; we want him to feel really stupid. Second, it has to have some feeling of being scary. And finally, we need to post this so everyone knows he fell for it. All agreed, we start out with a host of different ideas when someone brings up that there should be a way to scare him about an AIDS patient.

By this time, we have had a couple of AIDS patients in Chico, and you couldn't watch the news without some update or a new movie star or basketball player being diagnosed with it. We finally come up with the idea that somehow we need to get him dressed up as if he is going out to take care of some AIDS disaster.

We bring in the EMT that is working on the ambulance, and she is helping us organize this. We decide that we need to make up an AIDS package and have our target get dressed into it. But how? We finally contact the OR nurses, who are just as bored as we are, and they jump at the chance to help. We then contact central services and tell them we have placed a few things on the dumbwaiter and ask if they could wrap them then seal it in a package labeled, "Dr. Bowman's Memorial AIDS Package." They are a little hesitant, but after reassuring them that they won't get into trouble, they do it. We then have them send the package to surgery.

Now that all the players are in place, it is time to spring our trap. We talk one of the respiratory therapists into calling the dispatch line as we know our target would recognize our voices. Soon we hear the phone ring from the nurse's station, and as usual, we all start into dispatch to see what is going on. We can hear an excited voice on the other end of the line as he is telling Mark that he needs an ambulance immediately as he and his boyfriend have just been diagnosed with AIDS and his boyfriend can't take the thought of it and has cut his wrist. He then goes on to tell our poor dispatcher there is blood everywhere and that he thinks he's gotten the bleeding stopped, but to hurry. Mark hangs up the phone and is handing the dispatch slip to the ambulance EMT while telling her the story. She then drops the slip on the dispatch council, stepping back, saying, "No way, I'm not going!" In shock, Mark just looks at her, then says, "You have to go."

"No, I don't. I have a child at home, and I'm not going to bring this disease home." Then in a demanding voice she says, "You go!"

In shock, Mark has nothing to say, so we say it for him. "I think you'll need one of those new suits if you're going out to an AIDS patient." As he stares at us, still not saying anything, we start a conversation among the flight crew, ED nurses, and the ambulance paramedic. Mark is just standing there, not knowing what is really going on, new enough to know he can't refuse to do anything.

"I think those suits are kept in surgery, aren't they?" I ask.

"That's right, I believe they are," Mike replies, then asks the crowd, "What are they called?"

Everyone is kicking around different names when the charge nurse speaks up. "They are called the Dr. Bowman's Memorial AIDS Kit, I believe."

"Yes, that's it!" we all reply simultaneously.

We now can see a bit of a questioning look on Mark's face when the charge nurse tells him to call OR and tell them that he will need two of them. Hesitantly, Mark picks up the phone and calls the OR, thinking this is a joke and he will be making a fool of himself to the OR nurses. The OR nurse answers, and he sheepishly asks for the kit, then a bright, surprising look comes over his face when they answer back, "Okay, how many did you say you needed?"

Now totally hooked into the joke, he says, "Two, I need two."

"Okay, we will set them out at the window. You can just come down and pick them up."

Mark hangs up the phone and tells us that they will set them out, and the paramedic tells him, "I'll go get the ambulance pulled up while you go down to OR. Get the kits and have the nurses help you get dressed." He then turns and heads outside to where the ambulances are parked.

Mark, now just standing there, looks at us when Mike tells him, "You better get going. That guy is still bleeding out."

Mark runs to the OR, and as promised, there are two packages out on the window, sill just out of the OR. He grabs them, and when he returns, running down the hallway, he stops and asks us to help him get into one, as he has not been in-serviced on it yet.

Now, how great is that? You come up with a plan that is so good that the target of the plan is asking for help in getting dressed into the final phony outfit.

We can barely keep from bursting out in hysterical laughter, trying our best to keep as straight a face as possible as we open one of the packages. Still not knowing everything that the central supply people may have added to it, to our surprise, we find a full-size, bright-yellow, water-impermeable one-piece hazmat suit, a surgical hair cap with the cover for a full beard and mustache, goggles, pink booty covers, gloves, not surgical gloves, but a pair of way-too-large worn leather ones borrowed from someone on the maintenance crew, I'm betting. A really stupid-looking silver strap that we have no idea what to do with until Mike tells us that that is the belt and ties it around Mark's waist. And to top it off, someone has thrown in a vaginal speculum. We stare at it for a moment, all wondering what to do with it when Mike just grabs it and tucks it into Mark's new, shiny silver belt like a six-gun from the Old West. Now grabbing the second kit for his partner that is to go outside and pull up the ambulance, he shoves it under Mark's arm, points toward the rear doors, and yells, "Get going!"

Mark starts down the hall, and as he passes the remaining staff at the nurse's station that don't want any part of our plan, all bite their cheeks as he passes. Almost tripping over the pink booties and trying to hold the second kit from slipping with one of his over-size-glove-covered hands while the other is trying to keep the vaginal speculum from popping out of his silver belt, he passes through the automatic glass doors onto the outside ambulance dock, where he is greeted by roughly ten people from all the departments, OR, central supply, maintenance, respiratory, and the rest of the emergency department. All are snapping pictures of our stylish, new EMT as he is striding down the dock.

Shocked at all the flashes of cameras and laughter, he remains focused when, finally, roughly halfway across the street, and not seeing an ambulance running, it comes to him that he has been had. He just stands there in the street and turns to the crowd on the dock, who are all now clapping and cheering at him. He sheepishly pulls the full-face head-and-beard cover from his head, and we can all see the bright redness of his face as he slowly starts back up the dock, now bowing to the cheering crowd as he continues to pull the remains of the kit off and waving the vaginal speculum as if it is a trophy.

I think it takes us about half an hour to be able to stop laughing, and even longer to look Mark in the face without starting up again. Several of the staff from the other departments stay for a while to chat and laugh. All in all, Mark is a really good sport about it, knowing he has been had, and in true night shift tradition, he asks who would be next and he most definitely wants in on it.

For years, as I would pass through different departments in the hospital, I would see some of the pictures taken that night; they hung in most of the nurse's lounges in surgery and central supply as a reminder of that boring evening and that night shift rules! For years after that, my boss would tell me about a new EMT, paramedic, or nurse that was coming to night shift to finish their orientation, asking me, "Pease be nice. We like this person and would like them to stay for a while!"

17

A VALUABLE LESSON

EVERYONE WILL TELL you that in their career, they will learn many things, not only how to do things, but also how *not* to do things. I often tell students that if they ask five people how to do a specific procedure, they may easily get five very different answers in how to accomplish the same task. This can be related to the institution they went to school in, the instructor that first taught them the procedure, the preceptor that got them through clinical, or simply something they picked up along the way. In the end, many people, myself included, will either choose the one technique that works best for them or use parts of different examples and put them together to form a technique of their own. In the end, you will find a way to get something done that will seem the simplest and easiest way to you. Hence, *"There is more than one way to skin a cat!"*

There are also things you will learn in your career that will forever change the way you talk to patients. The biggest: Never make promises you can't keep. I'll never forget one of the most valuable lessons of my career, one that I learned as a paramedic and have passed on to EMT students, paramedic students, and nursing students throughout my career.

We arrive to work on a very hot evening, and as we are doing our preflight, we can't wait for the sun to go down and start cooling off. Jokingly, whenever it is over a hundred degrees, we always start talking about water and how we should have a call that includes getting wet, either wading in the river or out in the lake. Something to cool us off.

We finally finish our preflight, and even though we would love to stay up on the roof and chat some more, we know the charge nurse will be calling us soon, wondering where we are, and it is also just too hot to stand around up here.

As we ride down in the elevator and start cooling off, Bruce and I start pulling up our flight suits and wiping the sweat off our foreheads. When the doors open on the first floor, we step out and start down the hallway to the emergency department, stopping briefly at our lockers to drop off a couple of items, then continue down the hallway to check in and find out what we will be doing. As we approach the charge nurse, I can see my name written down in the treatment area and take a quick look at the patient board. Three out of four beds are occupied, and I can see that there is one arm laceration, one chest pain, and one LOL NAD (little old lady in no acute distress). I chuckle as I nod to the charge nurse, then disappear around the corner into the treatment area, stopping at the desk with the patient's charts. As I start to read the histories and try to get a grasp on what is going on, the nurse that is assigned to this area walks up and verbally gives me a report on what is happening, then asks if I could take over the college student with the laceration. She has just put him into the bed, and nothing has been done to him yet. I agree, and as I walk to the bedside to introduce myself to the young man, I ask him how he got the laceration. He then tells me that they were playing a softball game and he was the third baseman. The batter hit a fly ball into the area off the third baseline close to the fence and he decided to make a run for it. As he was running, looking up at the ball, he thought he had more room than he actually did and ran full speed into the chain-link fence and somehow cut his forearm. I smile for a second, then say, "Well?" He pauses for a few seconds, then asks, "Well what?" I let him hang for a few moments, then ask, "Well, did you catch the ball?"

His girlfriend, sitting in a chair next to the gurney and also wearing a softball uniform, the same team as his, smiles as I wink at her. The superhero ballplayer then sheepishly says, "No, I missed it."

A VALUABLE LESSON

"Dang," I reply, then add, "That would have been a super impressive play. You know, if you're going to end up in the hospital getting stiches, it would have been cooler if you had made the play."

The girlfriend then speaks up, adding, "Yeah, well, he actually did catch it, but after he bounced off the fence, he dropped it when he started screaming like a little baby."

"Ewwwwwww," I start, then add, "No sympathy here!"

I can tell the boyfriend wants to say something to defend himself, but one look at the girlfriend, who is throwing him a look as if to say, "Yes, you have something to say," and chivalry becomes the best answer in the long run and the boyfriend then looks back to me, changing the subject. He asks, "How many stiches do you think?"

Still slightly laughing, I give him the answer I give every patient. "It's a lot easier to count them after they are put in than before they are put in."

At this point, I have finished prepping the wound; it is numbed up, cleaned out, and I have placed the suture tray next to the patient on the stand. As I take my gloves off, I tell them that the physician will be in in a moment then sew him up, then I'll be back in to get them out of here.

I walk back to the nurse's station to chart what I have done as the ED doc comes into the treatment area and asks if the patient is ready to be sewn. I tell him yes as he walks into the stall and ask what kind of suture he wants. Pulling the gauze off the wound, he tells me to grab some 4.0 nylon. I step over to the cart and pull one of the packaged sutures from the box and open it for the ED doc to pull out with his sterile-gloved hands. As he is starting to suture up the wound, he asks the ballplayer how this happened, and I start to smile, wondering if the same story and verbal lashing will occur from the girlfriend. The man looks briefly at her then, turning to the doc, simply says, "I ran into a fence." Knowing the whole story, I chuckle a little, and looking at the girlfriend, I can see she is smiling and winks back to me, knowing she has whipped him down a little.

After the sutures are all put in, I clean up the wound and wrap it, and as I'm giving him his go-home instructions, including how and when to get the stiches removed, I can't help but run several comments through my head that I would like to tell him about his ball-playing career, ones that I'm sure the girlfriend would get a bigger kick out of than him, and just as I'm about to tell him maybe he should pursue a different pastime, maybe dominoes, my pager starts beeping.

Saved by the bell. I quickly have the man sign the paper and hand him his copy and thank them for a being good patient. Setting the paperwork down on the nurse's station, I tell the nurse that she can just leave it and I'll finish it when I get back. I see her nod as I round the corner and start a slow jog down the hall, listening to the pager. "FlightCare, scene call, boating accident west shore of Lake Almanor, heading zero one zero degrees, forty-five miles."

I reach the elevator just as the verbal finishes on the pagers, and find that Bruce has already called the elevator and is waiting for Tom and me. "Awesome!" the three of us almost say in unison, knowing we are not only going up into the mountains but to the lake. How cool is that?

As we reach the helicopter and buckle in, Tom is starting up the turbine and I am able to get more information from dispatch. They come back and tell us that there has been a boating accident, and at this time, they aren't sure where they are going to land us, as the patients are still out in the water or still in the boat. We acknowledge the information as Tom pulls power and lifts us off the helipad.

As we are heading to Lake Almanor, I know it is a very large lake, and the best dispatch can give us is that we will be going somewhere on the west shore. "Well, that's better than nothing," I answer. Working at the fire department on the other side of the lake, I am still somewhat familiar with the west side and explain what I know to Tom.

As we start down over the ridge, it is now dark, and we decide to fly to the lakeshore then start south, following it, thinking we should eventually be able to pick up some emergency lights. As we are making our turn to start down the shoreline, we suddenly get a call from the West Almanor Fire Department. After we answer, he fills us in that he will be setting up a landing zone in an intersection and thinks he can see us approaching. We ask him to activate his overhead lights, which he does, and we pick him up immediately. As Tom is slowing and making a recon circle, the firefighter in the rescue informs us that we will be getting in with him and he will take us down to the boat dock.

"Told you we were going swimming!" Bruce says with a smile, then adds, "We'll be thinking of you Tom, sitting all alone." He just giggles into the intercom, and as the skids touch down, the two of us pull our gear out, leaving the gurney, knowing that more than likely the ambulance crew will have our patient back-boarded. After tossing our gear into the back of the rescue, we jump into the front with the firefighter, and as he starts driving us the less than one mile to the dock, he starts filling us in on what he knows.

"Apparently, there was a ski boat with three guys and three girls in it. As they were boating back at the end of their day and it was getting dark, their judgment was somewhat impaired by the refreshments of the day and a combination of not knowing the lake very well, when they ran full speed into a solid rock formation about a half-mile off the shoreline. The boat slammed to a sudden stop, throwing everyone to the front. One of the guys was pronounced dead on scene, and another is in critical condition, and that is the patient they are bringing to us now."

"Damn, they must have been hauling ass," Bruce says, then follows with a question. "Why didn't they see the rocky island?" The firefighter then tells us that they have had several people hit it. Especially in the evening, the rocks are very dark, and when the sun is setting in your face, you simply won't see it.

"Wow, sounds like they should blast that thing out of there," I say, also knowing that I have seen this rock when I have been out on boat patrol with the fire department, but I really had no idea it was such a problem.

We arrive at the dock and can see other fire vehicles, an ambulance, and a couple of sheriff cars. We grab our gear and only guess that we are to go out onto the dock, as there is no one around. As we walk up to the crowd, we can see a boat approaching, and without asking anyone any questions, one of the firemen points to the boat and says, "Your patient should be in there."

ON THE GO

"Okay," I reply and watch as the boat comes closer, and finally, in the lights of the dock, we can make out the two ambulance crew and a firefighter taking care of someone in the rear of the boat. As they bring the boat up to the dock, one of the ambulance crew turns and, waving to us, yells out, "We can use your help!"

Bruce and I step into the boat and immediately notice that with the patient, driver, two ambulance crew and two firefighters, and a passenger, not only is the boat crowded, but maybe it's also close to being overloaded. I then politely ask if a couple of people could step out for a few minutes to give us some room. The two firefighters nod and step up onto the dock, along with the female passenger. As the ambulance crew starts giving us their report, I am checking the patient and don't really like what I see. He is moaning and combative. An EMT is trying to hold his arm somewhat still, but you can see that it is broken and bending in one too many spots. The man has an obvious head injury, and listening to his chest, I know he has several broken ribs and maybe a collapsed lung. I watch as Bruce is starting an IV and, knowing he needs to be intubated, finally decide to just get him out of the boat and I'll intubate him in the ambulance, where we have a little more control and better lighting on our ride back to the helicopter.

That decision made, we all put our efforts together and make sure the man is secured to the backboard, then lift him from the boat, passing him off to the firefighters on the dock, who then place him on the gurney and roll him to the ambulance. As we are doing this, I can't help but notice that the woman, not in ambulance or fire apparel, has been with us the entire time, and as they are locking the gurney into the ambulance, one of the EMTs asks if she can ride to the helicopter with us. Before I can ask who she is, he answers back, "She is his wife," pointing inside to our patient. I nod. "No problem. Just put her on the bench seat." I ask this knowing I want to intubate him and will need the seat at the head of the gurney for myself.

As I climb in and start pulling out the equipment I'll need for the intubation, I can see that the woman is very concerned about her husband. She isn't crying, and she isn't talking; she is just scared stiff.

A VALUABLE LESSON

Holding his hand in hers, she just keeps staring at him, and I can almost hear her frantic thoughts.

It doesn't take me long to insert the nasal tube, and by the time I'm securing it, the ambulance is coming to a stop near the helicopter and the rear doors open. As we pull the man out, the wife stays at his side, trying to stay out of our way but not wanting to let go of her husband's hand. It is quite obvious that they have a real loving relationship.

As we finally secure the man into the helicopter, hang the IVs, and start closing up the doors so we can start up and leave, I have to ask the woman to step aside. I gently take her hand from her husband's, and placing my other hand into hers inside of her arm, gently locking it in place as an escort would do, I start slowly walking her away from the helicopter, which Tom is now cranking up. When we are at the ambulance and I know I can leave her with the crew, I then ask her what the man's name is, and in a squeaky, scared voice, she answers, "Nick, his name is Nick."

Stopping at the ambulance and still holding her arm, I turn her around and tell her, "Nick is in good hands. We will be taking him down to Chico to the trauma center."

Now, almost afraid to let go of my hand, she manages a short, "Okay."

I then decide she needs one last thing before parting, and wrapping my other arm around her, I give her a hug. She almost immediately breaks out in tears, and taking an extra few seconds, I hold the terrified woman and tell her, "Don't worry, everything will be okay!"

I nod for one of the firefighters to come take over for me as I can hear the helicopter is now up to full RPM and I need to get going. I duck down and jog to the open door and climb in, and after pulling on my helmet and buckling in, we lift from the scene. Looking down, I can still see the woman now staring up at us, and I give her a wave as I close the door.

The trip back to Enloe is very busy for us, and one of the things you worry about in an aircraft while climbing in altitude is, if your patient has a collapsed lung, gaining altitude can change a simple pneumothorax into a tension pneumothorax, which can be fatal, making a bad situation worse. And in our case, it does. I can tell that the Ambu bag is getting harder to squeeze with each breath, and as I look at the monitor, not only is his heart rate climbing, but his oxygen saturation is also dropping. Bruce is watching this also, and we decide that his simple pneumothorax is now changing into a tension pneumothorax and he needs a thoracotomy. Bruce pulls the equipment out of the first-out bag, and while he is putting the syringe and equipment together, I wipe the patient's chest with a Betadine swab with my free hand. All assembled, Bruce locates his landmarks and slowly introduces the large needle into the patient's chest while aspirating on the attached syringe until the syringe suddenly fills with air. At that point, he slides the catheter in, and even though we can't hear any air escaping with our helmets on and the engine running, I can instantly tell the ventilations are easier, and by the time he attaches the Heimlich valve and we watch the valve working with each breath, the patient's oxygen saturation is slowly climbing and his heart rate drops back down to an acceptable rate. At about the same time, Tom has cleared the ridge top and is starting a slow descent to Chico. We know that as we drop altitude, the increased atmospheric pressure from being closer to sea level will also help our patient.

By the time we are approaching the helipad in Chico, all his numbers look good on the monitor, and just prior to landing, dispatch radios us to tell us that we have been requested back to the same location to pick up a second patient. We knew when we were there that there was the possibility of a second patient but didn't see him or her at that time; we figured they must have still been out on the wrecked boat.

We pass off the patient to the crew and slide in the second gurney. As this is being done, I ask Tom if he thinks he will need to take on some fuel to make another trip back to the lake, and he tells me that he has just been calculating that. By the time I buckle in, Tom is pulling power, and I can hear him telling dispatch that we will be heading to the airport to take on some fuel. Bruce and I then discuss a plan that he will stay in the ship and put things back together, and I'll help Tom out with the fuel.

A VALUABLE LESSON

As we touch down at the airport, we are at our spot next to the refueling trailer that the airport leaves for us so we can fuel after hours. I jump out of the still-running helicopter and run to the trailer, grabbing the nozzle and static ground cable, and, after flipping the power switch on, drag everything back to the helicopter. After I attach the ground cable, I take the fuel cap off and insert the fuel nozzle. Not being able to release my grip, I yell at Bruce to stick his head out and hand him the cord to my helmet. He plugs it in, and now I can talk with Tom while standing outside, fueling. After about three minutes, he tells me, "That'll do it!" and I stop the fuel, replace the cap, and kick the ground strap off the skid, which is on an automatic rewind, and as I watch it moving across the asphalt, building up speed back to the trailer, I follow it, winding up the fuel line, and finish by shutting off the pump. Jogging back to the helicopter, I can hear Tom is bringing it back to flight RPM and with one last double-check to make sure I've put the fuel cap on and it's secured, I climb in and give him a thumbs-up. We are airborne before I get my helmet plugged in again, and as I'm sliding the door closed, Bruce speaks up. "Well, that was the fastest refueling I've ever witnessed."

"Yeah, it goes a lot faster if you don't have to shut down and climb out," Tom replies.

Now restocked, refueled, and knowing where we are going, we all sit back in our seats and take a few minutes to go over the last patient and wonder about what our next patient will be. "That must have been one hell of a boat crash!" Tom says, and knowing he has a boat and that I have been out with him and his wife many times waterskiing, we finally come to the conclusion that it just isn't safe to be out on the lake after dark. Boats don't have headlights, and to make matters worse, a little alcohol and a little overconfidence in knowing where you are and where you are going can all add up to disaster.

As we crest over the ridgetop and start a descent to the lake, we make contact with the fire department and they tell us that the new patient will be brought to us and to land at the same place as last time. We acknowledge this, and in a few minutes, we are dropping down below the trees and setting down on the road.

ON THE GO

We can see the ambulance and decide to walk over to it and assess the patient before Tom shuts down. As Bruce and I climb into the back of the ambulance, I look around at all the people that are gathered and don't see the wife of the first patient. I want to let her know that all went well in our last flight. Turning my attention back inside of the ambulance, I can see Bruce is already assessing the patient and he is awake and answering all his questions. He is fully C-spined to the board and already has an IV hanging that the ambulance crew has started. After helping Bruce with a few of our monitors, we pull the patient out and roll the ambulance gurney over to the helicopter and slide him in. A quick wave to everyone, and Tom pulls power and we lift off the roadway, over the trees, and turn west back to Chico.

Bruce informs me that besides a broken arm and a few broken ribs, he actually looks pretty good. We monitor him and mostly talk about boating and skiing on our intercom en route back to Chico. As we land on the helipad, the ground crew walks up and we slide our patient out of the helicopter and start down the ramp to the waiting elevator. As we ride down to the first floor and the awaiting trauma team, the ED tech informs us that our first patient was taken to surgery and he believes he is still there.

We enter the trauma room and move the new patient over, giving a last-minute report and update. As I look around, I can see Drena in the corner and wink at her, which makes her smile. Bruce and I know we have a lot of equipment to grab and restock as well as two run reports to start, and looking at the patient board in the ED, I know the charge nurse will be bugging us to hurry up and get everything done so we can help them out. We decide that Bruce will go up and clean and restock the helicopter and I will start in on the paperwork. If I'm not done by the time he gets back down, he will try to help me.

I gather everything I need, face sheets, trauma sheets, billing sheets, dispatch records, my two-inch tape from both flights, along with a soda, then sit down at the computer. As I start filling in the forms, checking the checkboxes, and writing the narrative, Drena steps around the corner and sits down next to me. We start talking

A VALUABLE LESSON

about the flights and the injuries these patients have, and remembering that one person was killed, neither one of us has heard of such a bad boat accident.

As I'm starting my second run report, Bruce sticks his head around the corner and tells me that he is done upstairs and the charge nurse wants him to help out in the ED, then ask me if I need anything. I answer no, then tell him, "Matter of fact, I have already started on the second report and should be done in ten minutes or so." He says thanks, then disappears around the corner. About the same time, Drena's pager starts beeping and she gets up and steps around the corner to use the phone. I continue finishing the second report, and just as I am breaking it all down, she comes back around the corner. Instantly I can tell that something is wrong. Her face has lost its smile, and she looks very concerned.

"What's up?" I ask, not totally sure I want to know. Without saying anything, she sits back down next to me and, placing one hand on mine, looks me in the eyes and tells me, "That was the house supervisor. Your first patient from the boat accident just passed away in surgery."

I am shocked. All I can do is stare at her. I am at a total loss for words, and it takes me a few minutes before I finally ask, "What happened?"

"I really don't know, but I'll find out and get back to you."

My eyes are filling as I start thinking of the wife that was with us. I tell Drena about her and how she wouldn't leave his side, how she kept holding his hand, and then in one of the most idiotic moves of my career, I told her not to worry, that everything would be all right.

Drena wraps an arm around me as I bend over, holding my head in my hands. "Why did I say that?"

"Sometimes we say things not really knowing what the outcome will be."

"Yeah, but that was stupid," I tell her, then wonder how many times I have said that. How many times have I given people false hopes?

ON THE GO

Drena and I talk for a while, and knowing that the charge nurse will be hunting me down soon, we give each other one last hug before she heads off into the hospital and I go check in and start helping in the ED.

The boat accident call at Lake Almanor was a career-changing event for me. I have taught my heartfelt lesson to many students over the years, telling them to never make promises you can't keep, that destiny isn't in your hands, to tell patients, family, and friends of patients that you will do all you can and that is about the best you can promise anyone.

I still think of the woman I made the promise to and can only hope that over time, she has forgiven me for breaking my promise.

18

FOUNTAIN FIRE

"**Hey, Greg,** I need you to help out in the trauma room. A new patient will be here in about one minute!" the charge nurse yells at me just as I've entered the ED and haven't even had time to set my bags down. Looking up at the clock, I can see that my shift doesn't even start for another fifteen minutes. I usually arrive a little early in case there is a flight at the end of the day shift, so they can get home on time, but not to be thrown into the ED. As I stand there, contemplating on telling the charge nurse that I would rather go get my report from the day shift, exchange radios and keys, go check the ship, then report to the ED, I can see the charge nurse really doesn't care, as she has turned her back to me and is already talking to someone else.

"I hear you're with me!" I hear as I turn to see Pete, one of the ED nurses, who is also one of my friends.

"Yup, that would be me," I say, trying to add some enthusiasm as I walk into the trauma room and set my bags down on the counter, asking, "What is coming in?"

Pete starts filling me in as I am donning an x-ray apron. "All I know is that it is a stabbing victim coming from Oroville."

"Go figure!" I reply, knowing that most of the stabbings and shootings come from Oroville. "Anything more?" I ask, hoping to learn about the patient's condition, whether they are conscious, unconscious, breathing, or not breathing, but instead, all I get back is, "They say he still has a knife impaled in him."

Okay, I think. *This just might be interesting after all.*

I barely have my apron tied when I hear the ambulance pull up on the dock and a commotion coming through the back door. I peek out into the hallway and see the ambulance has brought an entourage of escort vehicles, including county sheriffs and city of Oroville police. I step back into the room and announce for all to hear, "Places, everyone! They're here!" Pete smiles, as he likes my way of bringing humor into some of the serious situations.

I can now hear the shuffling of feet and what I think is a squeaky gurney wheel and watch as the Oroville paramedics wheel the gurney into the room. There are also a couple of Oroville firefighters that have accompanied them in the rig, which in itself tells me that the patient may have been combative when they left town. As they push their gurney up alongside the ED gurney and start giving their report, I take a quick look at the patient, and besides his being covered in blood, I can see that he is in C-spine precautions, but a second look at the towel rolls next to his head don't make sense. Instead of the usual one towel roll on each side of his head with tape across his forehead and over the collar, there is one on the patient's left side, but two on the right, and they are not parallel to his head but perpendicular, ninety degrees to his head.

As we move all the IVs and the patient over, I listen to the report, and the paramedics are telling us that this patient was involved in a fight near one of the bars downtown, and according to his friends, about the time that he was winning the fistfight, the loser decided that he needed to take it to the next level or get his ass kicked. At this point, he pulled out a large knife, and after stabbing our patient a couple of times in the abdomen and chest, I guess he felt he needed to finalize the battle and rammed the knife as hard as he could into the patient's head.

As I listen to this, I can't help but lean over and look between the two towel rolls, and sure enough, I can see the handle of what appears to be a large knife sticking out of his head above his right ear. I then look up at the trauma surgeon, and when we make eye contact, I say, "Okay, I'm impressed!" The surgeon just shakes his head, and as we check vital signs, he orders an x-ray of the skull. After examining the wounds to his chest and abdomen, we ask him if he is going to be taking the patient to surgery. This would be the usual procedure for anyone stabbed in the abdomen, as they have to go in and look to see if any vital organs have been injured or control any bleeding, but in this case, our surgeon just steps back and, after thinking for a few seconds, tells us, "Call the neurosurgeon."

I now know he is thinking one of two possibilities: first, to punt this patient off onto the neurosurgeon, or two, that these wounds are not compatible with life and they should just let him expire.

As the x-ray tech walks back into the room with the film in his hand, all eyes are glued on the viewer, and when he flips the light on, the entire room fills with ten people simultaneously saying, "EEEWWW!"

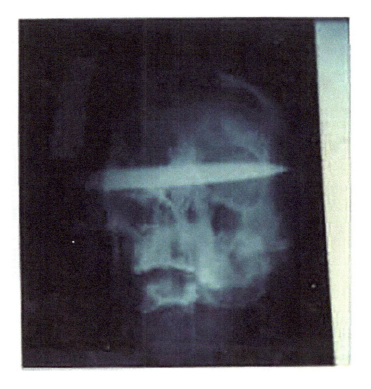

"I've never seen a knife that large traveling all the way across a patient's skull to the other side before," the trauma surgeon says.

Then I have to answer with a question of my own. "Has anyone in this room ever seen a knife clear through someone's head before?" I turn to see if anyone is holding their hand up, but all I see are wide eyes staring and commenting on the x-ray. No one answers, and now I can see that the sheriffs and Oroville police officers have joined us and are making comments of their own.

As we are joined by the neurosurgeon, the conversation starts up between him and the trauma surgeon, and they are trying to figure out what to do with our Buttant. The two of them finally come to the conclusion that the wound to the patient's head is a fatal injury, and even if his heart keeps beating, he will be brain-dead. The trauma surgeon adds that he believes he will succumb to his wounds in his chest and abdomen in the next thirty to sixty minutes anyway, and between the two of them, they decide not to take him to surgery and to just admit him to the medical floor and let him expire. As they are listening to this, the deputies and PD officers then ask, "We need the knife. It's evidence." The two surgeons then look at the deputy that has made the comment, and with somewhat of a smirk on his face—and you would only understand if you work with this surgeon—he tells the deputy, "Well then, pull it out!" Then he turns and walks out of the room with the trauma surgeon. The deputy then looks at me and, with a slight look of worry on his face, asks, "He was kidding, right?"

I think about this for a moment, thinking how much I really need to screw with these guys, and finally answer, "You want the knife or don't you?" Pete has caught on, and as he removes the towel rolls that are alongside the patient's head, now totally revealing the handle of the knife, he adds, "Here you go!" The deputies and PD officers then start into a conversation about not only what they should do now but also how they should do it. As I help with some details with the IVs that are infusing, both sheriff and PD officers walk up to me again and want to know if the doctors are kidding about them pulling the knife out. I turn to look at all of them at once, and as I am trying to think of something to say, something that will really mess with their already-scrambled minds, my pager goes off.

"Got to go!" I say as I untie and remove the x-ray apron. As I am hanging it on the wall hooks, the officers are still wanting an answer and are trying to stand in my way as my radio is announcing our destination. I finally have to force my way through, out of the room, and into the hall. As I start a slow jog down the hall toward the elevator, I take one quick look back toward the opening to the trauma room, and seeing several heads of lost law enforcement officers watching me jog away, I can't help but smile.

I reach the elevator, first calling it to the first floor. I can't help but laugh to myself, thinking of the officers and what they may be discussing. When Marty and Bruce arrive, they can see the smirk on my face and ask, "What's so funny?" Almost laughing, I start the elevator to the roof and tell them the story about the police officers wanting the knife that is sticking out of the patient's head and, after they said they wanted it, my telling them to just take it. Then jogging away and leaving them with a look of "You've got to be kidding?" on all their faces. As we exit the elevator and start a slow jog up the ramp, the look on the faces are still fresh in my mind, and I can't help but smile and laugh a little more, thinking that all those macho deputies and police officers are probably now drawing straws or roshambo to see who pulls the knife out, and in reality, knowing the patient will be expiring soon, they should just leave it and let the medical examiner deal with it.

I climb into the helicopter, and after fastening my belts, pulling on my helmet, snapping the chin strap, and pulling down the visor, I key up the radio and ask dispatch where we are going and what we are responding to. They answer me back with the latitude, longitude, heading, and mileage, then tell me that we are responding to a patient involved in an accident while trying to escape a fire. After a pause, I ask if this is also a burn patient, and dispatch tells us that most of the information is sketchy at best at this time. We tell them we will start that way and would appreciate if they would give us an update when it becomes possible.

Marty lifts the helicopter off the roof and starts a slow turn toward the north. As we gain altitude, I pull the map out, and as Bruce and I are looking down, concentrating on the map, trying to figure out where we are going, Marty suddenly gets our attention by saying, "I really hope we don't have to fly through that thing!"

Bruce and I look up from our concentrated job of map-deciphering, and in shock, both of us simultaneously let out an "Oh, shit!"

ON THE GO

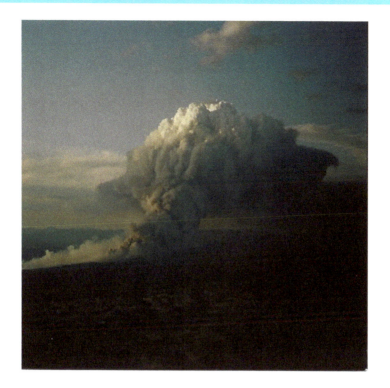

As we look out the front windshield, exactly in our path is an enormous smoke cloud from a very large wildfire. We double-check the map and keep looking up and finally tell Marty that we believe the coordinates they've given us are exactly where that fire is, maybe a little to the east, which we can see is the direction the fire is traveling.

We keep heading in the direction that the GPS is steering us to, and our hearts are pounding when dispatch finally calls us on the radio. "FlightCare, dispatch!"

"Go ahead, dispatch. This is FlightCare."

"Continue on your given coordinates. We have a different frequency for you. You will be flying into controlled airspace." He pauses a moment, then continues, "I guess there is some kind of fire near there and you will need permission to enter the area."

We look at one another, all thinking the same thing. *Yeah, right, some kind of fire!*

Dispatch continues telling us that after we are cleared in, we will be contacting a sheriff deputy on CALCORD but first have to contact Air Operations on an air-to-air frequency. Acknowledging this, we start dialing in the different frequencies into the radio.

As we get closer to the fire, we start picking up a lot of traffic on the air-to-air frequency and, when we are about ten miles out, can start seeing multiple large air tankers and helicopters working the fire. The different tankers are either dropping retardant or are in holding patterns at about one-thousand-foot-elevation intervals so they don't bump into one another. The helicopters are closer to the ground, and we can see different ones making water drops onto hot spots then returning to a reservoir to refill their buckets.

Marty has been waiting for a break in the radio traffic and finally decides that he either has to butt in or start circling. Keying up the radio, he calls the lead plane, which is also the Air Operations that is in charge of all aircraft, fixed-wing and rotor-wing, over the fire. "Air Operations, Enloe FlightCare on air-to-air." After a few more transmissions to different air tankers, the lead plane answers us. "FlightCare, Air Operations. What is your location and destination?" Marty quickly fills him in that we are approaching from the south at five thousand feet, and according to the coordinates given to us, we should be heading toward the far eastern side of the fire. The Air Operations plane then tells us to drop to one thousand feet and enter a holding pattern approximately five miles to the south of our destination. Marty acknowledges this and starts dropping the helicopter. Once at one thousand feet, and when we think we are about five miles south of where we are supposed to be, he enters into a big orbiting circle. At this point, we can see that we are now almost under the large smoke cloud, and as we look to where we think we will be going, the fire seems to be increasing in intensity, speed, and may already be there.

While we are orbiting, we decide to contact the sheriff deputy and switch over to CALCORD. "Sheriff 184, Enloe FlightCare on CALCORD." Immediately the deputy answers back, and we all can hear the anxiety in his voice as he is just short of screaming into the radio, "FlightCare, where are you? We need to get the hell out of here, NOW!" The urgency is unmistakable, and we tell the deputy that we are in a hold position about five miles south of him, waiting on a clearance to enter the controlled airspace. The deputy then keys up, yelling to us that if we don't get there in the next five minutes, the fire will beat us there and they will have to move to another landing spot, but due to deteriorating conditions and heavy smoke, they don't know where that will be. We try to distract him for a moment and ask if the patient is ready to be loaded as soon as we land. He tells us yes, that there is no ambulance here, only himself and one fire department rescue. They have put the patient on a spinal board and moved him to a field so he can be loaded.

The entire situation doesn't sound good, and after listening, Marty calls Air Operations again and tells him that we now understand that the landing location may be burned over at any time and we are requesting immediate clearance into the east side of the fire. After a pause, the radio keys up. "FlightCare, Air Operations. I have a visual on you and can see your landing zone. The fire is spotting nearby, and in that field, it looks like it won't last very long. Make your approach from the south, then exit to the east. There will be aircraft in all other areas and above you." Marty immediately pushes the nose over and banks the ship onto its side, making a very fast approach to the landing zone, at the same time replying to Air Operations, "FlightCare copies, here we go!"

As we fly in closer under the cloud, knowing we are only a few miles out, I slide the door open and the cabin instantly fills with smoke. As I turn in my seat and stick my head out the door, I can now see ash flying by, and as we get closer to the ground, red-hot embers are blowing by the aircraft on both sides. Some are swirling into the cabin. We make a slight turn around the thick cloud of smoke, and there, right in front of us in a field, we see the fire department rescue truck and the deputy car. Looking more to the left, I can see that the field is on fire, and it is now only about a quarter of a mile away and burning our way.

The landing in the field is nowhere near textbook or soft. Marty sets the helicopter down as if he is pushing it down, and even though he is telling us to go, he really doesn't have to. I don't even think the skids are on the ground when Bruce and I are out of our seats, hit the ground running, and race over to the rescue truck. We know if the fire gets too close, Marty will move or leave without us and that we may have to just hang on to the back of the rescue as it races out of the field.

We reach the rescue truck, and with only a quick look to see that the patient is unconscious, and after listening to the EMT tell us that he has been this way since they took him out of the truck that he was driving when he hit a tree, we quickly decide that is enough of a report. Then, just as I am about to tell everyone that we need to go, movement catches me out of the corner of my eye, and looking up, I can't believe what I see.

As I take a quick look to the west to see how close the fire is, suddenly bursting out of the flames is a horse running directly toward us, and he is running as fast as he can. His fur is totally on fire. We all watch in disbelief as the poor animal runs by us within a few yards, whinnying in pain and catching more of the field on fire as his burning fur falls from his body.

Moments after the burning horse runs by, we hear the unmistakable sound of rotor blades. Looking up, I see a large bucket coming out of the smoke and then see a helicopter attached to it. The bucket seems to open up at that exact moment and looks as if the water is going to drop right on us, but with the forward momentum of the helicopter, the water drop lands exactly between us and our helicopter, putting out a few of the small fires the horse has started and paving a wet path for us back to Marty.

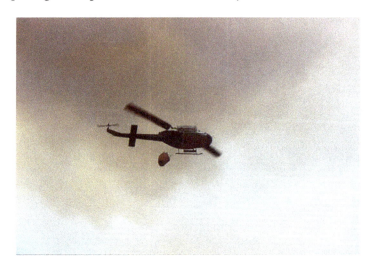

ON THE GO

"LET'S GO NOW!" I yell and, without waiting for anyone to answer, lift one corner of the board, and with everyone also knowing we now only have seconds, we run to the running helicopter and literally throw the patient onto the flight gurney. Not taking the time to fasten any straps, Bruce dives in, and I jump into my seat, snapping my lap belt. Before I have my helmet plugged in, Marty is already pulling up on the collective. I take a quick look in the field and can see that the sheriff and fire truck are now racing out of the field, dirt flying from their tires, and when they get to the fence line, they don't even slow down and just drive through the barb wire and onto the roadway.

I slide the door close, and looking out the windshield, I can see that Marty is flying only feet above the ground, trying to stay under the cloud of smoke and watch as hot embers are bouncing off the windshield. Neither Bruce nor I are looking at our patient. At this point, it is all about personal survival. If we don't make it out of here, we will be doing no favors for our patient. We need all eyes outside. Marty has the helicopter at full power, and now, at over one hundred miles per hour, the ground is moving under us remarkably fast. After what seems like an eternity but I'm sure is only seconds, we can see that the cloud is lifting and we have made it out from under it. The three of us sit back in our seats when we hear the radio. "FlightCare, Air Operations. Are you still in there?" We know the lead plane probably lost sight of us when we flew in under the smoke cloud, and when the horse caught more of the field on fire, we are sure he might have thought that the fire had caught us on the ground.

Marty keys up the radio and calls, "Air Operations, FlightCare."

Answering back, we can tell the pilot in the plane has been a little worried about us. "FlightCare, Air Operations. Where are you?"

"We are airborne, flying east. We would like to make a turn to the north to continue to Redding, if that is okay with you?"

Now more relaxed, the lead plane calls back. "FlightCare, Air Operations. Okay, I have a visual on you now. Go ahead and make your turn. Stay under one thousand for five miles, then you are clear." There is a pause as Marty is making his slow turn to the north when the radio keys up again. "FlightCare, glad you guys made it out of there. You had me a little worried."

Marty then keys the transmit button, answering him, "Yeah, we were a little worried ourselves. Thanks for that water drop. It made a big difference."

Air Operations then tells us to have a nice day, and Marty replies the same to him.

Now out of the fire area and away from the multiple aircraft circling the fire, Bruce and I suddenly realize that, hey, we need to take care of our patient! We have been so focused on getting in and then out from the fire that we have almost forgotten about our trauma patient. Doing a good exam inside a running and flying helicopter isn't the best place to get this done, but if you take in the other option, staying on scene longer and maybe burning up, this isn't so bad.

The patient's head is between my knees, and I can see that he has several contusions and lacerations from head wounds that I can only think came from his truck hitting the tree, and more than likely, he was not wearing a seat belt. As I study his level of consciousness, Bruce continues to assess him from the neck down to his waist. I place an oral airway into the patient's mouth not only to help hold his airway open but also to assess his conciseness further. And as I thought, the airway slips in without any change in our patient. At this point, and looking out the windshield, I can see that we still have at least fifteen minutes to Redding. As I start pulling the intubation equipment out of the bag, Bruce fills me in that the patient has a large contusion on his chest, and when he palpates his chest, he can feel several broken ribs. He also tells me that his abdomen seems to be fairly firm and his pelvis seems to be intact. As far as his extremities, we both know he has a broken left arm as we can see that the fire department has just tucked it under one of the straps but his hand is still twisted around backward. As far as his legs, they look straight and we don't see any bleeding, and we will just leave them alone. In reality, there isn't much in the way of a threat to one's life from having a leg wound as long as the patient isn't bleeding.

Bruce takes a second look at the left arm and finally decides to just leave it alone. He still needs to start a couple of IVs and place the patient on the cardiac monitor, pulse ox, and blood pressure machine. While he is scrambling to get this done, I have pulled out all the equipment I need to place the endotracheal tube and slip it into place without any difficulty. As I am securing it and hooking it up to a bag valve mask, I take another look at the pulse ox so I can have a base reading in case the patient starts developing a tension pneumothorax from the positive-pressure ventilation of me assisting his respirations.

Before we know it, Marty is approaching Redding and lets us know that we are less than five minutes out. Bruce has finished placing all the equipment on the patient and, totally impressing me, has two IVs running and taped down. Sitting back into his seat, he pushes the Transmit button and starts giving the hospital a report on our trauma patient.

I take a moment while squeezing the bag to look out the window as we are flying over the city, and I can see Mercy Hospital on the hill. I used to work here part-time, and it truly is a beautiful facility. I remember being totally impressed with the way the hospital was set up, especially taking advantage of being on the hill, as they attempted to put as many rooms and offices in locations that overlook the city. The dining room for all the staff is a combination of indoor and outdoor dining. You can stay inside if it is raining or 120 degrees outside or go out and sit on the balcony.

We circle the hospital from the north and make our approach to the helipad that is on the ground level and outside the emergency department. As we approach, I can see the Mercy helicopter sitting on the pad and the trauma team standing a safe distance off, waiting for us to set down. I slide the door open to watch for any loose debris as Marty gently sets the A-Star down, a far different and softer landing than the one in the field at the fire.

After the skids set down, Marty throttles back the engine, and as I step out and wave the team up, they walk up to us, bend over, all wearing hospital scrubs and x-ray aprons. We slide our patient out onto their gurney and start our walk to the hospital and into the ED. When we arrive in the trauma room, I give a quick report on the patient and what we know about the accident and what we have done for him en route. One of the doctors asks if he was restrained or if the fire department had to cut him out of the truck, and I simply tell him, "I really don't know. We didn't have much time to get a full report." I decide to not go into the details of the fire, the burning field, and the burning horse running by. In fact, I don't think they would believe me anyway.

I toss a couple of items onto the gurney, and the two of us push the gurney out into the hallway. I ask the ED tech if he has something I can clean the gurney off with, and he steps around the corner to grab some towels and spray. As we are wiping things down, I see the Mercy helicopter crew walking up, pushing a gurney of their own. We start into a conversation with them and then walk out with them to the helipad.

As both crews are putting items back into their own ships, we joke around about the different calls we were on. They tell us that they've just brought a patient that is a direct admit to the ICU from the smaller hospital in Weaverville, then ask us what we have just brought in. Bruce, Marty, and I just smile, and finally, Bruce asks, "Do you think they will believe us?"

"Nope!" I reply, then look at their faces and can see an interest in hearing what this is all about. Now knowing it is over a hundred degrees in Redding and must be another twenty degrees hotter on the helipad, I suggest we go to the cafeteria for some cold drinks and we will fill them in while sitting in the air-conditioning.

It doesn't take any convincing to anyone that this is a good idea, and we all stroll into the hospital and down to the cafeteria. As we grab some cold drinks, the Mercy fixed-wing crew also joins us, and soon we find ourselves pushing a couple of tables together to fit all of us. For the next fifteen minutes, we tell our story. By the time we finish with our story, we can see that there must be another ten or fifteen people leaning over, eavesdropping. Most of these people are sitting with their backs to the large windows, facing us, and finally, one of them asks, "How big do you think this fire is?"

Looking over his shoulder, I raise my hand, pointing out the window, and tell him, "Take a look for yourselves."

They all turn around and, in astonishment, can see the very large cloud of smoke that is now resembling a mushroom cloud from a nuclear bomb that is visible for at least a hundred miles. In unison, many of the doctors, nurses, and paramedics all let out with an "Oh, shit!"

Soon, Marty, our timekeeper, is standing up and telling us that we need to go. We still have to fly out to the airport and fuel up, then head back to Chico. After topping our sodas off, the Mercy flight crews all walk out with us to the helipad, and we say our goodbyes. Marty fires up the ship, and we lift off to transition over to the airport, which is only about a mile. I just leave the door open for the short ride. By the time we finish fueling, it is dark out. We lift off and start flying south along Interstate 5, following the stream of headlights for most of the way until we reach Red Bluff, then branch off to the east, now following Highway 99 to Chico.

As we are starting over the city and can make out the helipad light on the rooftop. Marty starts an approach to the hospital, flying down our well-rehearsed path, trying to stay over the Esplanade and not fly over any of the homes in the area. Then, just as we are slowing and making our last final approach to the rooftop, now only about thirty feet from landing, dispatch calls us, telling us not to land, that we have a request to Chester. Marty pulls up on the collective, and pushing the nose over, we fly over the helipad only about fifteen feet above the roof. Looking down, I can see the people in the parking lot looking up at us as we clear the far side of the roof, and I think we may have scared some of the pedestrians.

Chuckling, then sitting back in my seat, looking out over the lights of the city, I key up the intercom. I comment, "Well, I think it's going to be a busy night."

19

MEDICAL LEGAL

"**IF SOMEONE IS** refusing medical care and you continue to treat them, can you be sued?"

"Good question. Anyone want to take a shot at this?"

I really enjoy teaching the medical legal portion of any of the first responder, EMT, or paramedic classes. I can always stimulate a good conversation in the class. And as with this question, if you can be sued, it worries a lot of students. In reality, the answer is simple: yes, you can be sued. Come on, this is California. You can't go to the bathroom without running into a lawyer waiting for someone to slip on the freshly mopped floor to give out his card. I usually shock the students with that answer but follow up by telling them, "Yes, you can be sued, but the better question is, Will it go to court or will it stick?" I then go into lengthy discussions and explanations of the following. "For an emergency worker to be successfully sued, they have to prove several things."

First, *Was there a duty to act?* Are you properly trained, and are you on duty? If so, yes, you have to do your duty and do the best at what level you are trained for. If you are a volunteer and decide not to respond because you're having a birthday party for your two-year-old, do you have to respond? As long as you didn't sign up to be on call for that time and, as such, this would leave the ambulance or engine unattended, then no, you don't have to go.

I then give them this scenario: If you are driving along on your day off, in your own car, and you come upon an accident, do you *have* to stop? The class will usually open up into so much interaction that I usually have to tell people to raise their hand and we will call upon them in turn. After a lot of discussion about why you should or are required to stop and why you should just keep on driving and let the paid people handle the situation, I give them my best answer. First, if your car has fire department and EMS stickers all over it, someone is truly injured, and the bystanders see this advertisement on your car, you could possibly be held accountable to stop and help. I'm sure the people with their cameras on, taking pictures of the people bleeding on the highway, will snap a picture of your car and ask authorities why you didn't stop.

Personally, I use *the Greg stand-up rule*. I drive by the accident slowly, and if everyone is standing up, looking okay, I keep on driving. I can always argue that everyone looked okay when I passed by. If someone is trapped in the car or lying on the ground, yes, I'll stop.

The *Good Samaritan law* protects the common driver, encouraging people to stop and render aide, knowing they won't be eligible for a lawsuit. But for a trained individual that does this all day long, the law can get a little fuzzy. For instance, if an off-duty EMT stops at the same scene, happens to have an IV set up in his trauma bag he carries in his personal car, and decides to put in an IV in this patient yet starting IVs isn't in his scope of practice, and the eight attempts sticking expired needles into the patient's arm end up in an infection and amputation of the patient's arm due to this infection from the failed IV start, or the three litters of IV fluid he infuses puts this patient into congestive heart failure and then they spend two months in the ICU because of the overload of fluid and complications from the amputation of their infected arm and, in fact, the only injury from the accident was a twisted ankle, then no, the Good Samaritan law isn't going to help you.

Next, *neglect*. Could you have done something that would have either saved this person's life or helped in some way? Yes, if you are there and choose to not help the individual because he smells bad, has spit on you, or has called you a bad name but he still needed care, yes, you have neglected him. This is one of those fuzzy parts of the Good Samaritan law. If a trained paramedic is spotted driving by this same accident and is not stopping and it is proven he could have done something with his knowledge and saved the driver's life with only what he had on him or in his car, then maybe.

Third, do no harm. If you purposefully further injure this patient in the course of your treatment *and* it was done purposefully with the intent to inflict pain or harm, yes, you are a candidate for a suit. But, at times we inflict some pain that can't be helped—starting an IV is painful, manipulating a severely broken leg that is wound around the car's brake pedal is painful, but it cannot be helped if we are going to get this person out. On the other hand, dropping the gurney with them on it down a flight of stairs? Okay, I think you get my point.

Lastly, refusing care. "If a patient refuses care and I continue to treat them, can I be sued?"

"Maybe!"

There are a lot of answers to this question. First, is the patient a minor? If so, they cannot refuse. The courts look at this as, "The prudent parent would want their child treated and transported to a care facility without waiting to get the parents' permission." Or is the patient drunk or impaired? This is one of the worse questions, as we have to ask, "How impaired are they?" We have no idea most of the time, and in fact, usually it is best guess at the time of the incident, and falling back to the same answer as the minor, the court will look at it as *implied consent*. Were you trying to help someone that may not have been in the proper state of mind to make correct decisions for themselves?

One of the perks of being an instructor is, I get to tell stories and the students have to listen, and this is where I like to put in one of my favorite stories to tell the students.

"It was a dark and stormy night. Don't laugh, it really was!"

Clay and I are grounded from the helicopter because of the weather and have talked the charge paramedic into putting us on an ambulance. After a lengthy discussion, a.k.a. whining, he only agrees if we are in the rotation and take whatever call comes up, making a point by telling us, "Not only the traumas, medicals, or out-of-town transfers, but if there is a call to the nursing home to transport a ninety-nine-year-old with no bowel movement for two weeks and somehow this has become a medical emergency at two in the morning, we would have to go, understand?" Grudgingly we accept. Not exactly what we want to do, but any chance to get out of the ED would be okay. I guess we have to take the good with the bad.

Part of our deal also is that we would get the first call of the rotation, and it isn't long before we are paged out to a private residence to treat a seventy-year-old male with a chief complaint of shortness of breath. Clay, our EMT, and I handle the call without any problems, and when we get back, we pass the charge paramedic in the hallway and jokingly say, "You're up!"

After unloading our patient on one of the ED beds, restocking the rig, and finishing the paperwork, the two of us go back to work in the ED, taking care of different patients, hoping we will get out again tonight but know the other crew is up. A couple of hours pass before we hear the pager going off for the other crew, and I stop what I am doing to listen and hope I'm not going to miss a good call when the audible comes out. "Medic 2, respond to Oak Hill Convalescent Hospital for an eighty-three-year-old female with a urinary infection. Time out, zero one twenty-two."

I almost wet my pants laughing when I hear this, and before I can breathe, I see Clay peeking around the corner from a patient's room, laughing. Then I hear someone behind me speak up, asking, "What's so funny?" I turn to see Drena, and she can see that tears are welling up in my eyes and I'm holding my stomach. Once again, she asks, "What?" I finally catch my breath enough to tell her how the charge paramedic has said Clay and I could be on the rig tonight if we agree to take whatever call comes up and how he's made a special point of telling us, "Not just the good ones, and if we get paged for some old guy who hasn't had a bowel movement in over two weeks, we would still have to go pick him up." Funny thing is, now he is going to pick up an old woman with a chronic UTI.

Drena joins me in my laughter, and we start into a conversation about some of the more colorful transports the ambulance has to make sometimes, and even though administration complains about improper transports, there never seems to be an alternative solution. I then tell her how I had picked up an elderly lady once that wanted a ride to the doctor's office but we had to stop at the grocery store first, then the pharmacy on the way home.

Clay has joined us and starts to tell us a couple of stories of his own from his time working as a paramedic in the Bay Area when, midsentence, he is interrupted by our pagers going off. The three of us stop talking, holding our breaths, crossing our fingers that we don't have to go get the constipated man in the nursing home, when the audible comes over the radios. "Medic 4, motor vehicle accident, car into a building, near the corner of Broadway and Second Street, time out, zero one forty-three."

Clay and I look at each other for a split second before we turn to start a jog down the hallway, but as I attempt to leave, I feel a tug on my sleeve. I turn to see Drena looking at me, and with a worried look, she says, "Be careful, please!"

"No problem" I reply, wink, then head down the hallway and out to the ambulance. The EMT already has the rig fired up before either Clay or I arrive, and I jump in the back as Clay is climbing in the passenger side of the cab.

Our EMT turns on the red lights and starts out of the parking lot and, when he turns onto The Esplanade, flips on the siren. From the location they've given us, this accident should only be about five or so blocks away, and because the speed limit through this part of town is only thirty miles per hour, we aren't expecting much of an accident, but this is still better than the convalescent home and the constipated man.

The three of us are joking and laughing, thinking how pissed the charge paramedic will be when we get back, and of course, I have to throw in my favorite quote about being pissed off. "You know what I always say, better pissed off than pissed on!" We all laugh.

Our laughter is cut short when we hear the first Chico fire engine arrive on scene and give a report of a single car into a building and they are requesting heavy extrication equipment and two more engines. This puzzles us, why is all this extra equipment is needed. We are driving code 3 and are only doing around thirty-five to forty miles per hour.

As The Esplanade rounds the corner into the downtown area of Chico, it splits into two one-way streets, Main and Broadway.

Broadway is the street we will be on, headed south, as Main is the one-way returning north the opposite direction one block away. Broadway also makes somewhat of a left bend as it enters the downtown area, and as we are entering this turn, we can see the fire engine, other police vehicles, and a lot of people standing on the sidewalks, watching. As we pull in closer, the three of us are dumbfounded. There is a car almost halfway into a solid redbrick building. The front of the car is destroyed, and it looks as if it's struck the building right in the doorframe of the main entrance. I know this building and know it is a restaurant and can only hope no one inside is injured.

As we exit the ambulance, a police officer walks up to us and quickly tells us that no pedestrians or patrons in the restaurant were injured, but witnesses state the car was traveling at a speed of around eighty miles per hour when it entered the bend in the road and couldn't make the turn. "Did you say eighty, like eight-zero, eighty?" The officer nods, then continues by telling us that there are two people trapped in the car.

Clay and I nod at each other and know that we will split up, each taking one side of the car, and check out the two patients. As I'm walking up to the driver's side, I look down and can't help but notice an enormous amount of coins scattered all over the road and sidewalk. It suddenly dawns on me that these are probably coins out of the parking meters, and with a quick glance down the sidewalk, I can see several of these bent over and a couple just gone.

I arrive at the driver's side of the car, and I can see and hear the driver yelling and telling the officers and firefighters that he is okay and to just leave him alone. I can also see that his left upper arm is broken so severely that not only is it a compound fracture with the bone sticking out, but he is also oblivious to this and is waving it around, trying to push the fire personnel away from him. The nearly detached forearm is flailing around wildly. I take a quick look over the top of the car at Clay and tell him I have a critical, and looking back at me, he tells me the same. I then yell at our EMT to call for a second ambulance. We know that we will be taking these patients one at a time as we get them extricated.

I push my way through the firefighters that are trying to talk sense into the patient, but he is having nothing to do with it. I know

MEDICAL LEGAL

the firefighters need to get to the task of getting the jaws out and start cutting this car apart so we can get these patients out, and I ask if one of them can stay and help me, knowing our EMT is trying to run equipment back and forth to Clay and I, both with our own demands, and somehow he is keeping up with it.

Because the patient is awake and cussing at me for trying to take care of him, I know he is conscious, but maybe not totally cognitive of what is really happening. There is a strong smell of alcohol coming from the car, and I can see a laceration to his forehead where he hit his head on something. I know because of the alcohol and his head injury, there is no reasoning with him, so I just go about my job of trying to take care of him and simply agreeing with everything he is saying, with a, "Yes, yup, okay, you want to go home. Okay, whatever you say." The firefighters have caught on, and we have finally caught the broken arm that is waving its bones at us and showering us with blood. The arm is nearly severed completely off, but to my surprise, I can still feel a pulse in the wrist.

The fire captain has told both Clay and I that they are going to have to free one side at a time and think they can get the passenger side open first. I acknowledge and can also see the second ambulance has arrived, and the charge paramedic is asking where he can help. We tell him to help Clay, as his patient will be out first, and they can start him into the hospital. We also ask him to radio the ED and tell them we will be having two trauma activations. He nods and does this as he moves over to Clay's side to assist in getting his patient out. My patient's side of the car is somewhat under a large pile of bricks that came loose during the impact, and the fire department is having to move some of them off the car and from around it so they can make room for the extrication team to come in with the jaws as soon as they are finished with the other side. I also notice that the other engine companies have arrived, and with the added personnel, things are starting to fall into place and move along a little faster.

Between the three of us, we get our patient's arm somewhat stabilized, but one of the firefighters is having to physically hold it so the patient doesn't toss it around any further, possibly loosening it from its temporary splint. I have managed to start an IV in the other arm, and there is a firefighter in the rear seat attempting to hold the patient's neck in C-spine precautions. I have been able to do a little more exam and can tell he has many broken ribs and decreased lung sounds on his right side. I really can't judge his abdomen very well, but looking at the bent steering wheel and seeing that he isn't wearing a seat belt, I'm betting he has internal abdominal injuries. At this point, I have no idea about anything below his waist, and it won't be until we get him out that I can really assess that. Amazingly, this entire time, the patient is insisting that he is okay and wishes we would leave him alone and let him drive home. Not one word of pain or wondering why all these people are gathered around him or why they are cutting his car open like a can of tuna.

Clay has left in one of the ambulances with his patient, and I ask the charge paramedic, who is going to ride with him, to return after dropping Clay and his patient off at the hospital, as I may need an extra hand. Although the fire department is working as fast and as best as they can, the problem is complicated with the fact that they think the building may be somewhat unstable. It is an old three-story building, and they don't want to do any type of movement to it. They finally come up with a plan and ask me if it is okay. They want to hook up to the car and pull it backward, away from the building, so they can get better access to the driver's side, and then they can cut it apart better. "Sure, why not!" I say, as if I were going to say no.

Soon they have a cable and winch hooked to the rear of the car, and just as they are starting to pull, the second ambulance has returned, and the charge paramedic walks up to me, asking what is going on. I fill him in on the plan, and as we watch the car being removed from the building, we can see more bricks falling, which is a little unnerving, but can finally see the entire car as it is pulled out over the sidewalk and onto the street.

When the winch is done, the firefighters jump on the car and start ripping into it. Before long, the driver's door is off and they let me look inside for a moment while they reposition the jaws. I can see that both of the patient's legs are broken. His left leg is so severely broken that not only is the femur protruding, but his tibia and fibula are both protruding as well. It is literally a tangled mess.

MEDICAL LEGAL

The firefighters finally have the steering wheel pulled out of the way, and it looks as if we are finally going to be able to get our patient out. We slide a backboard under his butt and, with a "One, two, three," slide the driver out and onto the board. While we are securing him onto the board and then rolling him on the gurney to the ambulance, he is still trying to convince us that he is okay, and I finally agree with him and say we are just giving him a ride home. I see no reason to argue, knowing he isn't going to remember any of this.

I jump into the back of the rig with the charge paramedic, and the two of us start attaching the patient to the equipment in the rig and start a second IV. After cutting the patient's remaining clothing off, the charge paramedic points to the patient's twisted legs and asks if we should do anything with them. Looking at them, I finally answer, "I am not even sure which way to turn them to straighten them out. I think the less we manipulate them, the better at this point." He agrees and knows that when we get to the hospital, the orthopedic surgeon will help with that before he goes to surgery.

The ambulance is now screaming through the streets, heading back to the hospital, and the patient is still oblivious to anything going on around him or to him. I radio a report in to the hospital, and in just a few short minutes, we are pulling up on the back dock. We quickly pull the gurney out of the rig and roll the patient into the trauma room and report off to the team.

The charge nurse has also asked if I can stay and help out in the room, and I agree. I start by helping the x-ray technician take x-rays of the patient as the trauma surgeon does his evaluation. He puts a catheter into the right side of the patient's chest to reinflate his collapsed lung and is very concerned about the patient's abdomen. As the x-ray films come back, the tech starts putting them up on the viewer. There is a film of the patient's leg on the viewer, and after studying it for a moment, twisting his head to one side, then the other, the tech pulls it off and rotates it 180 degrees. We all turn around to look at the patient's legs, then back to the x-ray, trying to figure out which way is up or down, right or left, but the leg is so broken and twisted it is almost impossible to tell. The orthopedic doctor takes one look at it and shakes his head, knowing this is going to be a long day in the OR. We then fill him in on the splinted arm and how the patient was flailing it around and how it looked to be nearly severed off but still had a pulse. The ortho surgeon reaches down, grabs the patient's wrist, and feels the radial pulse; all the time, he never stops shaking his head. Finally, after a few moments of thought, he asks, "Where did you say this happened?"

"Downtown, Second and Broadway."

"Really, downtown? This looks as if it happened on I-5."

The trauma surgeon tells us he wants to take the patient to surgery to do an exploratory laparotomy as he thinks the patient has some type of bleeding in his abdomen. The orthopedic surgeon only nods and says he will be along in a few.

I watch as the ED tech and OR nurses roll my patient down the hall to the surgical suite, thinking to myself, *You never know what you may find with this job.* I feel a nudge and look to see Drena bumping into me. "Hey, how's it going?" I ask, as if I don't know.

"Just fine." She doesn't have time to talk and needs to follow the patient to surgery, but as she smiles in passing, she shakes her head, saying, "I just don't know how you find all these patients."

I can only smile and shrug my shoulders.

I notice the charge paramedic walking back into the hallway after putting the rigs together, and before he can say anything, I ask, "If my math is correct, I think Clay and I are back up on rotation?"

Shaking his head, he answers me, "You've got to be kidding me. I don't know how you manage to get calls like this. I am always stuck with the UTI from hell, and you get cars into buildings."

"What do you want me to say, luck of the draw?"

We all laugh and discuss the call for a while, and soon the day shift is walking through the door.

We join the day crew in the break room, and they ask if we got to do anything last night. Clay tells them that we were put on the ambulance for the evening, and when they jokingly ask if we got anything besides bowel obstructions, Clay and I look at each other as if to ask if we should tell them about our call or not. I finally tell them, "Yes, we had an MVA downtown." They automatically think it was some type of low-speed fender bender or something in a parking lot and go about their morning routine as if it isn't worth having a conversation. Neither Clay nor I feel any need to tell them more as we are sure by the time we return tonight, they will have learned more and will be full of questions.

Back to the class. I now ask my students if they understand the scenario I just gave them, using it as an example of when it is okay not to do as the patient asks. Reviewing the different choices one by one, I explain each of them. First, *duty to act*. We were on duty, trained in these situations, and had a duty to act. Second, *negligence*. We were obligated to take care of this patient regardless of his request. It would have been neglect if we didn't take care of him, as he was not understanding his injuries, and because of his head injury and intoxication, he fell under implied consent. Third, *do no harm*. Obviously, the manipulation of his broken arm and twisted legs was going to cause the patient a lot of pain, and we did manipulate them knowing this, but it was done with good intent, as we knew we had to straighten them out or unwind them lose from the pedals of the car to get him out and save his life. This was acceptable. Fourth, *refusal of care*. Everyone on scene could hear this gentleman refusing care and just wanting everyone to leave him alone so he could go home. Because of his head injury, orthopedic injuries, and intoxication, there would not have been a judge in the state that would let this go to court if he attempted to sue us for not abiding by his demands and treating him regardless of his wishes, knowing that he more than likely would have died if we had left him alone. Explaining that even though the patient was adamant about not needing any care, he obviously needed it.

Courts stand behind EMS workers, as they know we are often put into situations like these. That there would truly have to be a documented case of neglect, undue harm, and the patient would have to prove they were not altered by alcohol or a closed head injury and making rational choices that a normal person would make before they will even hear such a case, wasting their time.

20

TRIP TO SACRAMENTO

"**I NEED TO GET** out of here," I tell Drena. It is around one in the morning, and she has come down to the ED to deal with some case that I'm not involved with but decide to check up on me while she is here.

She knows I'll be wanting out of here as the helicopter has been down due to weather for the last three nights. Mike, my scheduled partner for the evening, has already beaten me to any chance of going home early. He called in before his shift and talked the charge nurse into letting him off for the evening, and Tom did the same, telling dispatch to keep an eye on their monitor of the helicopter on the roof. If they start seeing the radio tower in the monitor behind the helicopter, which is a mile away, they are to give him a call, but as it stands right now, not only is it intermittently foggy, but it is pouring rain, a double whammy for me to not go anywhere. Unless there is a critical care transfer that needs a nurse to go by ground.

"I need some help in bed 2!"

Our heads automatically turn to the yell for help, and my body is already starting a slow jog, rounding the corner into the treatment area, when I hear, "CLEAR!" I arrive at the foot of the bed just in time to see the patient landing back onto the gurney after a defibrillation has passed through her chest. The nurse is now looking at the cardiac monitor and, at the same time, yelling out orders for us to do. "Someone start bagging her, someone grab some lidocaine, and I really need an IV!"

"I got the IV!" I yell out into the assembling team of ED nurses, techs, RT, and doctors.

As I'm grabbing a couple of angiocaths and an IV start kit from the code cart, I can hear the nurse now filling in the doctor that she had just brought the woman back into the room from triage. She had been complaining of chest pain, and just as she attached her to the monitor, she went into V-fib. She quickly shocked her once and now has a rhythm and pulse back. I am now kneeling down onto one knee along the patient's left side, with her arm dangling from the gurney, with an IV tourniquet on it, preparing to start the IV. As I scan the arm, choosing my vein, I can hear others going about their jobs. One nurse is drawing up medications and wants to know if the IV is started yet, the respiratory therapist is ventilating the patient with an Ambu bag, and the tech is flooding the IV for me. I have picked my site and give it a quick wipe with an alcohol prep then quickly advance the needle, and just as I'm advancing the catheter into the vein, I hear a strange gurgling sound.

At that point, the entire world suddenly has changed into slow motion. I am holding the catheter in place, knowing it is very important not to lose the IV, as the patient needs medications to stabilize her heart, but at the same time, in a very slow, loud voice, I can hear the nurse at the head of the patient that is helping the RT yell out, "She is going to puke!" and with that, I see her turning the patient's head to the side, my side. "NOOOO!" I yell out as I see the slow motion of stomach contents leaving the patient's mouth and coming right at me. I only have a fraction of a second to turn my head before feeling the warm, chunky, slimy, stinky goo hitting the side of my face. Instantly I can also feel it landing on my flight suit and running down the inside and starting to soak through the entire right side all the way down to the tops of my boots.

"Oh my god, I am SOOOO sorry!" the nurse says in shock of what has just happened.

I slowly turn my head back and look up at her, only able to open my left eye, as I can feel slime on my right dripping down onto my cheek. "You know, sorry just isn't going to do it," I say as I attach the IV and tell the tech to finish taping it down.

ON THE GO

I grab a couple towels off the cart as I pass by, walking over to the sink. I turn it on and completely dunk my head into the flow of water. As I pull my head out and reach for a towel, I notice someone is handing one to me and, with my good eye, look and see Drena holding out the towel, biting her lip.

"Don't even think of laughing," I tell her, but that is all she needs and she bursts out laughing, trying to talk at the same time but can't. As I stand there trying to dry my hair and pull more chunks out, she is now holding her stomach and leaning onto the counter. Knowing she can't talk, I then ask if she wouldn't mind going to surgery and grabbing me some scrubs. Now only nodding, she starts down the hallway and I yell out one more instruction for her to bring them to the lounge.

Now totally disgusted, I wrap the towel around my neck and head to the lounge to disrobe and jump into the shower. By the time I reach the lounge, I have taken inventory of my suit, and as I'm pulling items out of the different pockets, I notice that the two pockets on my right side that were open, are now full of vomit. I empty my books out of my suit onto the table, kick off my boots, then step into the shower, fully clothed. *Why not?* I figure that the best way to get all the vomit off my suit and out of the pockets is to just jump in. With the water running, I unzip out of my suit then hold it under the running water and reverse the pockets that are loaded with what resembles to be potato soup. When I am finally satisfied that most of the chunky stuff is rinsed off, I drop the suit onto the tile floor outside of the shower and turn my attention to cleaning myself off. As I'm trying to rinse out whatever is in my right ear, I can't help thinking that the nurse turned the patient's head toward me knowing I was down there, then finally I realize, she probably didn't see me squatting on the floor.

As I shut off the water and reach for my towel, I hear a knock on the door. "Who is it?" I ask, knowing that is probably Drena, returning with my scrubs.

"Scrubs are us," she answers back through the door.

"Just a second," I answer as I am finishing drying and wrapping the towel around me.

I open the door, reaching out for the scrubs, seeing that she is holding them out in front of her for me, but just as my hand reaches them, she turns her arms away to her side so I can't grab them, telling me, "I am not sure if these will fit. I might have to take some measurements or help you choose the right ones."

I smile, looking at her with a big smile on her face, telling her, "Just give me the scrubs." She slowly turns her arms back toward me, and I'm able to pull the scrubs out of her arms. "You're really funny, but you didn't have to laugh at me when I was covered in puke," I tell her as I pull on the scrubs.

Now laughing again, she continues, "Couldn't help it. I haven't seen anything that funny in a long time."

"Yeah, I'll remember this. You owe me."

We continue to laugh and talk as I finish drying my hair and she hands me a brush to comb it. Just as I am thinking I should either grab her and throw her into the shower or give her a big embrace, the lounge door opens. "You about done in here?" It's the charge nurse, wanting to know if I can finish up and come back out to help.

"Yeah, just finishing," I say as I wad up my flight suit and stuff it into a plastic patient-belonging bag that Drena has brought.

I catch Drena's eyes once again, and with a shrug of the shoulders, knowing that the hug will have to wait, the three of us leave the lounge and walk back up the hallway.

As Drena and I are chatting, we hear the ambulance going out to some type of vehicular accident and possible fire. The two of us slowly wander over to the radio to listen as we hear the ambulance and fire units responding. As the first engine arrives on scene, they report that there are two vehicles involved in the accident and one of them is on fire. Within seconds, the level of the radio traffic intensifies as we hear there are still a couple of people trapped inside the burning car. Shortly after that, the ambulance arrives on scene and radios back to us that the fire department has knocked the fire down and it appears that one of the two people in the burning car is dead and the other is still alive but trapped and it may take about thirty or forty minutes to get them out. At the same time, the second ambulance has arrived and will be bringing in two patients from the other car that is involved, but neither one of them seems to be critical, and they feel that they don't need to be trauma activations.

We fill the charge nurse in that there will be a trauma as soon as they get the remaining patient extricated and they think it will be in about thirty minutes at the earliest. The charge nurse then asks if I can take the trauma, as I am not going to be flying tonight, not only due to the weather, but also because now I don't even have a flight suit. So at this point, I'm an ED nurse. I agree and walk into the trauma room to give it a good look over. As I enter, I turn the speaker in the room up a little so I can monitor what the ambulance is doing and go about setting out a few items the physician may need. About fifteen minutes later, the ambulance calls in to let us know that they will have the patient out and be en route in about another five minutes. The charge nurse takes the report then calls the hospital operator to have them page the trauma team. As I hear the overhead page, "Trauma team in five minutes," I put on my x-ray gown, and at the same time, the ambulance is calling in their report.

"We have a thirty-year-old female who was the trapped passenger in a two-car motor vehicle accident. She was trapped in the burning car. She is currently only moaning with pain, fractures to her right arm and right femur. She has second- and third-degree burns to possibly 80 to 90 percent of her body. Vital signs are as follows."

The crew takes a break from the report, and I take a look at Drena, who has been standing with me, listening. We both know this doesn't sound good, and if she survives, she may need to be transported to UC–Davis's burn center. The crew then comes back with the vital signs, and in reality, they don't sound too bad. "Heart rate is 100, BP is 128 over 76, and respirations are around 16." They also tell us that they have her on high-flow oxygen, one IV running wide open, and they are starting a second. They also suggest having paralytics available to intubate her upon arrival. After hearing this, I walk over to the airway drawer and start pulling out the intubation equipment just as the respiratory therapist (RT) arrives, and seeing me pulling out endotracheal tubes, he turns around and heads back to his department to grab a ventilator.

The trauma physician arrives, and I start briefing him on what is coming in, and he asks me if I would go ahead and intubate her if she needs it after she arrives. I tell him no problem, and when the trauma nurse arrives, I ask her if she would push the paralytic medications that I already have out on the stand so I can be in position to do the procedure. She agrees, and as the rest of the team arrives, we brief them on what is coming in until we hear the ambulance calling in that they are about two minutes out.

We all fall into our positions, which most of us have gotten used to over the years. The lab people know where they should be to get a quick blood draw, the x-ray team has already placed a film in the slot in the gurney to get a chest x-ray, the ED tech knows he will be helping move the patient over, hanging IVs, and undressing the patient of any remaining clothing, the RT will be at the head of the gurney to help me, then take over with the ventilator, and finally, standing in the corner with the OR nurse, waiting to see if the patient will be going to surgery, will be Drena, taking notes, taking possession of any valuables we remove, and helping us try to not only identify the patient but also get ahold of any family.

As the ambulance crew comes through the door, almost immediately I close my eyes and turn my head as my nose picks up the horrible smell of burnt flesh. As the smell passes through the room, you can almost see the wave as it hits each nurse or technician, and they do the same, some holding their sleeve up over their nose.

We move the patient over to the gurney, and as the physician starts his exam, the woman only moans to any painful stimuli he inflicts onto her. Before he goes any further, he turns to me and simply tells me, "Go ahead." I know exactly what he means, and having the instruments I need in my hands, I nod for the nurse to push the paralytics. Within seconds, I can tell the patient has become nonresponsive and paralyzed. The RT has started ventilating her with a bag and mask, and when we both feel comfortable that we are ready, he lifts the bag and steps back. I insert the laryngoscope blade and, within a few seconds, have the tube in place, and the RT is hooking it up to a ventilator. I step out of my current position at the head of the bed and start checking the running IVs and watch as the ED tech is trying to remove what clothing is left on the patient. He has cut away what's remained of her blouse and bra, and we can see that there are burns all over her chest. As he is trying to pull away her pants, he is suddenly faced with a problem and looks up at me for guidance. I look down and see the woman had been wearing pantyhose under her pants, and they have melted to her skin. The two of us then slowly pull away the pants until we are both looking at her legs and waist. I try to pull some of the melted pantyhose off her legs, but each time I pull, layers of burnt skin try to peel off as well. We finally look at the physician, who has been watching us, and he asks, "What do you think?"

"Well," I say, taking a pause, then finishing, "I think we are only going to do more damage trying to get these off. If you really want my opinion, I think we should leave this job for the burn team at UC–Davis."

"Excellent idea!" he says, then turning to Drena, he asks her, "Can you get me Davis on the phone?"

Drena gives him a nod as she goes out to the nurse's station to call Sacramento. The trauma physician then tells us that he really can't find much wrong with her except the broken arm and leg and that her major injury is the burns. He then tells us to bring him the lab work when it comes in, splint the arm and leg, and if the x-rays and labs are okay, we will be moving her to the burn center at UC–Davis. I nod and start in with the tech, making plaster splints for her arm and leg, then decide I should let the charge nurse know she will be moving to Sacramento.

As I start explaining this to the charge nurse, she tells me that she has overheard the trauma physician and is already planning on it. Knowing I want to do the transport, I stand there like a dog wagging my tail, not barking, but hoping for a treat. The problem is, the charge nurse knows this also and wants to screw with me. She turns to the board and starts going through the names of the nurses on the board, pointing to each name, one by one. "Let's see, she can't go, she will be going home soon." She points to another. "Maybe he can go. He likes doing transfers. No, he told me he needs to be home on time. Humm!"

"Okay, I get it!" I exclaim, then ask, "What do I have to do to buy this transfer? You know I'm the only field nurse you have on tonight, and I'm one of the few that won't be on overtime." I really don't have to sell myself, and the charge nurse knows I'm the only one that can do the transfer, but that doesn't stop her from messing with me. She then, without a word, circles my name and writes "TX UCD" next to it. "Cool, thanks," I say as I step back into the room and, picking up the phone on the wall, call dispatch, letting them know I'll be in need of an ambulance for the transfer. They acknowledge, and before I turn from hanging up the phone, the physician walks back into the room and tells me that he has the lab work back and everything looks okay. He will write some orders for the transfer, and we can leave when we are ready. Drena has heard this, and I see her walking to the recording nurse to help with the arduous job of copying all the paperwork, labs, and x-rays.

As we are finishing with the paperwork, the charge paramedic walks into the trauma room and asks me if we need a whole crew to go. He then tells us that they have been really busy tonight and really don't want to send an entire crew on a five-hour transfer if I can manage the patient in the back by myself, as he can call in just an EMT to drive. I look at the patient, and knowing she will be paralyzed and I can place her on the ventilator from the helicopter, I tell him, "Yes, I'll be fine with just a driver."

"Okay, give me about fifteen minutes, and we will have a rig and driver on the ramp for you."

"Perfect!" I tell him, knowing that we will need about that much time to prep the patient and have everything copied.

As I get the patient ready for the transfer and gather enough medication for the two-hour trip, Drena has finished copying the paperwork and tells me that she will continue to try to get ahold of some family of the patient and let them know we are on our way to Sacramento. As I'm making one last check of the items I believe I'll need, my EMT walks into the trauma room with the charge paramedic pushing the gurney. He has come over to help us load up and send us on our way.

We transfer the patient onto the ambulance gurney, and after we roll her into the ambulance, I take a moment to get the ventilator up and running, the one that I borrowed from the helicopter, and make sure my monitor leads are still attached and I have a good EKG rhythm. The pulse oximeter is attached and working, the Foley catheter bag is hanging on the side of the gurney and urine is slowly draining into it, and finally, both of the IVs are dripping at the rates I want.

"Okay, I believe we are ready," I tell the EMT, and as he steps out the back, Drena sets all the paperwork down on the back of the bench seat and, looking up at me, pauses, then tells me, "Okay, you're all set. Please be careful."

I take a look back at her and wink, telling her, "Don't worry, I'll be fine!" just as the doors slam shut.

The driver jumps in the front and asks me if I'm ready, and I tell him, "Yes, let's go." I want to tell him to be careful with the rain-soaked roads, but I know this EMT and know he has been around a while and has lots of experience. As he pulls away from under the awning on the ambulance dock, I can hear the rain starting to hit the windshield, then the rest of the rig. A quick look out the front windshield, and I can see that not only is it pitch-black out, but it is really pouring, and the wipers are barely keeping up. As we round the corner, leaving the hospital, I hear the siren coming to life on the front of the rig and we start our code 3 trip to Sacramento.

Turning back to my patient, I look up and notice that one of the IVs seems to not be running correctly, and as I'm studying the drip chamber on it, I feel the all-too-common bump in the road as we cross the Esplanade. Then suddenly I hear the driver yelling, "SHIT, HANG ON!"

As I attempt to reach out and grab onto something and try to turn to look at what he is looking at, I feel the brakes being slammed on, and *WHAM!* Something slams into the passenger side of the ambulance. Because the impact is on the passenger side and I am sitting at the head of the gurney and hadn't had time to grab onto something and not wearing a seat belt, I am violently thrown against the side door and then down into the well of the steps. As I'm lying there, I only hope the door doesn't open and I end up on the street. Before I can reach up to pull myself out of the steps, a second series of big bumps bounces me and every piece of equipment in the back of the ambulance up and down a couple of times. With each bounce, my back is slammed to the floor onto the metal steps that I have landed on. A few seconds after that, I can tell that the driver has finally been able to bring the rig to a stop.

"You okay?" he yells from the front.

As I pull myself back upright and take a quick look out the front window, I answer, "Yeah, I think so. What the hell happened?"

I am surprised when he tells me, "A truck hit us. I have to jump out and see if he is okay."

"Okay, I'll check my patient. Let me know if you need anything."

As I sit back down in my seat, I can hear the driver calling in the accident on his radio, then hear dispatch toning out Chico Fire, Engine 2, and I'm really surprised when they answer back that not only are they already on scene, but the wrecked ambulance is in their front yard as well. Hearing this, I look out the window again, and sure enough, I can see the open engine bay doors; the engine is still parked inside, and the firefighters are just walking out to help us out. I also hear an ambulance being dispatched from the hospital and know this won't take long, as we are only across the street. We haven't made it one block before the truck has hit us.

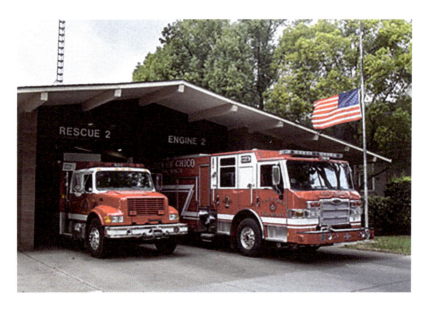

I quickly look over my patient and see that she is still secured onto the gurney and the ventilator is still functioning, as it's been clamped down. The cardiac monitor wasn't as fortunate, as it wasn't strapped down and is now on the floor. I also find one of the IVs that was hanging from the ceiling lying on the floor. I grab the IV and, double-checking it, find that it is still in good shape and still running. I hang it back up on the ceiling, then lift the cardiac monitor up and place it back onto the bench seat and find that the handle is cracked where it wasn't before, and all I'm seeing on the screen is a flat waveform. I really don't believe that the patient's heart has stopped, so I start checking the leads and find that two of the four electrodes has been torn loose from the patient in the impact. After I apply new electrodes, the waveform returns to the monitor and I study it for a minute, as it doesn't look quite the same. Finally, I figure out that even though the thing is working and reading the patient's heart rhythm, the screen is missing about an inch of its display on the left side. I whack it a couple of times with my hand, thinking that maybe it will return to normal, and after the second whack, I notice the screen is now missing about one and a half inches of display. "Better not do that anymore," I say to myself as I straighten up a few more things that have come dislodged in the accident.

One of the back doors suddenly opens, and I see the charge paramedic sticking his head in, asking if everything is okay. I tell him that the patient and I are okay but the cardiac monitor may be a trauma activation. He looks at me with a funny look, and knowing that I don't really want to take this conversation any further, I ask him, "Is this rig going to be able to continue the trip, or are we going to have to switch out?" He then tells me that the entire passenger side is caved in and we are going to have to move the patient over to his rig. I really don't want to move the patient and all the monitors, IVs, and ventilator, especially in the rain, but it sounds like it really isn't a decision I get to make. The paramedic then tells me that they will be pulling up next to us and will pull their gurney out and just transfer ours into their rig.

"That sounds good." I reply, then add, "Can we hurry this up a little? This girl really needs to get to the burn center!"

"I'm on it," he replies, closing the door, and soon I hear the second ambulance pulling up alongside us.

By the time I get the patient ready for the move, the rear doors open, and between both crews, we are able to transfer my patient out and into the new ambulance without getting too wet. As I'm now setting up in the second ambulance, the charge paramedic asks one last time if I need anything, and looking around, I suddenly realize that I don't have my paperwork. He runs to the first ambulance and grabs all the paperwork and x-rays, then sets them on the bench seat. With a final "Good luck!" and with a stupid smile on his face, he closes the door before I can reply.

The EMT that has come with the second ambulance will now continue with our trip as the first one needs to stay and talk to the police and document his side of the story of the accident.

We start out for the second time and, within a few minutes, have hit the freeway and start our trip, leaving Chico. Knowing I still have about an hour and a half, I keep a close eye on the patient, whom I'm keeping paralyzed. I have a few comments with the driver but don't want to distract him as he is driving in this torrential downpour, and I decide one accident a night is enough.

By the time we are passing through Marysville, which is about halfway to Sacramento, I notice that the screen on the cardiac monitor is getting smaller and smaller. It seems as if someone is slowly closing a window from the left to the right. *I wonder, if I turn it off and let it reset, will it return to its previous full screen, or is it possible that it won't turn back on at all?* I decide to just leave it alone. I only hope I still have something on the screen when we reach Sacramento.

The rest of the trip is pretty much uneventful. I keep up with the vital signs and make sure the oxygen saturation is maintaining good numbers then, feeling the brakes coming on, look out the front window to see we are slowing and leaving the freeway on the off-ramp to the medical center. I get one last set of vital signs, and as I'm unplugging all my equipment, the driver is backing into one of the ambulance parking spots. He hops out and opens the rear doors and has asked one of the other Sacramento ambulance crews that are standing around to give us a hand unloading. This they do without any problem, and we thank them.

ON THE GO

Now with everything tucked into the gurney or being held by the two of us, we start into the busy emergency department. The charge nurse spots us, and she gives me a funny look, as if to say, "Who are you, and what are you doing here?" Before she says anything, I tell her that we are a direct admit to the burn unit. She nods, and as we push our patient through the busy hallway, everyone stops to glance at our poor, burned patient. I have forgotten about the smell, as I have become accustomed to it over the last several hours, but looking at everyone's face, I can tell they are hoping we just quickly pass through and don't stop.

One of their ED techs has seen that we are a little overloaded with equipment and paperwork and has offered to help us up to the burn unit, and the charge nurse agrees. We enter the hallway, and as we roll up to the elevator, there are already several other people standing there, waiting for it. By the time it arrives and the doors open, we push the gurney in, and the ED tech, holding the door open, looks up at the people, who have not made any attempt to get in, and says, "Come on in, there's room." All the other people just shrug their noses and, in unison, say, "We'll catch the next one." The tech lets the doors close and, after they do, turns to us and says, "I didn't think they would, but it was fun to ask."

We arrive at the burn unit and report off to the staff of physicians and nurses. They take our report as we are all moving her over to their bed. The physician wants to know how much fluid she has had and when was the last time I gave any medications. I brief him up on all this, and finally done, we leave the burn unit and head back to the ED. When we arrive, the tech grabs some cleaning items and helps us clean the gurney before we put it back into the ambulance. Not wanting to smell the remains of the burned patient's skin that is still visibly stuck on the dirty Enloe linen, I decide to donate it to the medical center and toss it all into their hamper.

Knowing that there is pretty much no restaurants open on the way back to Chico this time of the night, we decide to put everything into the ambulance and go down to the cafeteria and grab a sandwich and soda for the trip home.

Now, sandwiches and sodas in hand, the two of us jump into the rig and start our trip back north. The EMT asks about the accident tonight, and with him knowing I had been in another accident while in the back of an ambulance years earlier, the conversation is pretty much about different ways to crash ambulances and ways to get hurt on this job. I think all the talk about crashes and injuries finally affects me, as by the time we are passing back through Marysville, I am starting to feel the results of tonight's accident. I find myself having a hard time sitting in the seat and can't seem to find a position that is comfortable. By the time we are pulling up on the ambulance dock back at Enloe, my shift has officially ended about an hour ago, and all I can think about is getting home, downing some Tylenol, and going to bed.

I am tired, and by the time, I shower and finally hit my mattress. I'm totally worn-out. The events of the night have been very stressful, and I go right to sleep. When I awaken around noon, before I even try to roll out of bed, I know something isn't right. Any movement and I feel pain in my back. With much effort, I'm finally able to get up and find that trying to stretch it out only seems to intensify the issue. I spend the next couple of hours downing Tylenol and ibuprofen, hoping that I'll feel better before I go to work again for another night. By midafternoon, I finally decide that I'm only kidding myself and decide to call my boss and tell her that I don't think I'm going to be able to work tonight.

After I get through to her, she tells me that she is glad I've called. She has heard about the accident and is worried. She tells me not to worry, that she will take care of covering my shift, but since this is a work-related injury, I need to come in and be seen as an ED patient.

Not really wanting to do that, I try to talk myself out of going in, but she won't listen to any of my wimpy excuses and finally tells me that she will start checking me in now and all the paperwork will be ready by the time I get here. I hang up the phone with a silent "Shit" and finish putting on some clothes. I find it fairly hard to bend over enough to put my shoes on and finally manage with the use of only one hand.

ON THE GO

The bumpy ride in my four-wheel-drive truck really isn't much fun, but I manage. As I pull into the parking lot, I can see a few people standing next to the area where the ambulances are parked, talking and pointing, and as I slowly drive by, I can see they are pointing to the damage to the passenger's side of the rig I had been in. After parking and walking into the back door of the ED, I'm greeted by my boss, who is waving me back to the clinic. As we enter, I see she already has a room saved for me, and I thank her for not making me wait in the waiting room with all the other patients. As she is taking my vital signs and after I have put on a hospital gown, she takes a look at my back, and with an "Oh, that must have hurt," she tells me that there are really wide abrasions and bruises running across my back where I must have bounced on the steps when I was thrown to the floor of the ambulance. As she is finishing her nurse's notes, she pulls out a large stack of paper and, handing me a pen, tells me that this is all the incident reports and work comp paperwork that I need to fill out about the accident and about my injury. I don't even get to argue the point as she smiles and leaves the room.

The head of the gurney is up at about a forty-five-degree angle, and I am able to lie back, put my feet up onto the bed, and use my legs as a desk to start on the forms. Before too long, the ED physician enters, and as he shakes his head, the first thing he says is, "This isn't your first ambulance accident, is it?"

"No, I've been down this road before, but this is nowhere as bad as the last one."

Interested, he then asks, "What injuries did you have from the last accident?"

"Well," I start, "I had a fractured pelvis, abrasions on my face, and my back was covered in road rash."

"Wow, I didn't know you had been ejected," he says, surprised about the road rash. Then I fill him in. "Well, I actually wasn't ejected. I was pinned to the top of the ambulance when it was sliding down the highway upside down and the roof tore away." He only lets out a small laugh, shaking his head.

After checking me out and seeing the big bruises on my back, he asks about them, and I tell him that I was thrown down into the steps of the doorway in the collision then was bounced up and down a couple of times as the ambulance jumped the curb. He decides to order some x-rays of my back to just make sure I didn't mess anything up and, looking at all my paperwork, tells me that it looks as if I have plenty to do to keep me occupied until they come for me.

After he leaves the room and I start back on the paperwork, I hear the door opening again. I look up over the top of the paper and see Drena peeking into the room. "You decent?" she asks.

Smiling, I answer, "Yes, come in."

"Darn, I really was hoping you weren't decent," she says with a bigger smile. She comes into the room, and as she gives me a hug, I let out a small grown as she squeezes me around the chest.

"What?" she asks.

I sit forward in the bed and point to the back of my gown. She sets her clipboard down, grabs my gown, and opens it up further to reveal the large bruises and abrasions on my back. "Holy shit! That must have hurt!" she says as I slowly lean back onto the gurney. "I heard you were only in a fender bender and continued on to Sacramento."

"Well, yes, sort of," I say, then continue, "We had to transfer to another ambulance. That one wasn't roadworthy anymore."

"I had no idea," she says, now placing her hand on my leg. "Are you going to be okay?"

"Yes, I'm going to be okay. You know me, I bounce pretty well. Give me a week and I'll be chasing you around up and down the halls."

This brings a smile to her worried face, but I can tell she isn't happy about it. Before she can say anything more, the x-ray tech walks in and wants to take me to his department. Drena tells me to make sure I check back with her before I leave, and getting up slowly from the gurney, I tell her that I will. She then gives me a much softer hug as I turn and leave the clinic and walk down the hall for the x-rays.

After the films, I walk back to my room and finish all the paperwork just as the ED doc and my boss come walking into the room. "Well, Doc, what do you think?" I ask. Not really saying anything, he motions for me to sit up in bed and starts feeling my back one more time, and I can tell he is looking for something. As he is slowly palpating each of my spinal vertebrae, I ask, "What are you looking f—"

At that moment, he hits a spot that makes me jump up, stopping me midsentence.

"Does that hurt there?" he asks, knowing that is a dumb question, or I wouldn't have jumped. He doesn't wait for an answer, telling me, "There is a questionable deformity on the film that shows you may have a small compression fracture in your thoracic spine."

"What? Are you shitting me?" I ask.

He then goes on to tell me that he will have the film reviewed by a radiologist and he may want me to follow up with an orthopedic surgeon.

Knowing I don't want to be put on the injured list, and looking at my boss, who has joined us in the room, I ask when he thinks I will be able to return to work. He tells me that he would like to have the reviews from the orthopedic and radiologist but then asks when I am scheduled to work next. I tell him that I have three days off until I am scheduled again. He then offers to give me a week off, and I finally come to a compromise that if I feel better in three days, I'll come to work. My boss knows that I will be here regardless, even if I am still not feeling well, because that's just who I am. We agree, and he writes my go-home instructions with a prescription for some pain medications. As he leaves the room, my boss has me sign the instructions and asks if I am going to have the prescription filled.

"Hell no!" I tell her.

"I didn't think so, but you should consider it just so you can get some sleep tonight."

"I'll think about it, thanks." I sign the discharge, and she gives me the paper, and I hand her all the paperwork she needs for me to fill out.

As I'm leaving the room, I pick up one of the phones from the nurse's station and page Drena. I wait around a little bit, and she doesn't return the call. Knowing she is probably busy, I gather my things and head out to the parking lot and climb into my truck.

After making a quick stop to grab something for dinner, I return to my apartment. As I flip through the channels on the TV, I finally give up around three in the morning and go to bed.

A couple of hours later, I am awakened by the faint sound of the front door of the apartment opening. I lie there listening, trying to make sure that is what I've heard, or maybe it's one of the other apartment doors. Then I hear my bedroom door opening. Lying on my side, I open one eye and can make out a familiar silhouette slowly coming through the door and making its way around to the other side of my bed. Without turning over, I lie there, listening, when I hear a zipper slowly being pulled down and the unmistakable sound of clothes dropping to the floor as the covers are being lifted and someone is sliding into the bed behind me. Now filling my nose with the sweet smell of Drena's perfume, and without turning around, I ask, "I hope you're not a burglar?"

I smile as I feel her cuddling up behind me and sliding her arm around my chest when she answers, "No, I'm not a burglar. I'm just the serial rapist you've been reading about in the paper." After a gentle hug, she then asks, "What am I going to do with you?"

Placing my hand on hers, I squeeze it, then reply, "I'm not sure, but this is a pretty good start."

21

HOME AT LAST

IT HAS BEEN a long, dark drive returning home from the game in Maxwell. The drive up the Feather River Canyon at night is not only dark but also windy, hilly, and very deserted. As I drive along, I can point out to myself all the different spots I had landed in the helicopter to help with some tragedy and try to save someone's life along with the fatalities we left behind.

Mile after mile, story after story, memory after memory. Sometimes I think it is a blessing; sometimes I think it is a curse. I'm not saying I have a photographic memory—my high school teachers will confirm that—but when it comes to the many calls I have been on, once I recall the actual incident, I can picture the most minute detail, what I found when I got to the patient, what the car looked like, what we had to do to treat them, and their transport back in the helicopter. This has proved to be very helpful in my life teaching different EMS classes, as I can throw scenarios at the students from my memory. I have also found it a curse when something triggers a call that maybe didn't go well. Maybe we didn't save that patient or child. I can still see the terror permanently etched into their faces.

As I see the lights of Portola glowing in the distance, I know our trip is almost over. A quick glance over my shoulder, and I can see that all the boys in the back seat of the Ram are still fast asleep, as well as the boy in the front passenger seat. I simply don't know how they can sleep on that windy road, but I guess they are simply exhausted after a long day and a very hard fight for the win at the basketball game. I guess having them sleep far outweighs any possibility of them

HOME AT LAST

having car sickness, which we have had in the past returning from games, but not tonight.

As I slowly come into town, I am suddenly running different scenarios in my head on how I should wake up the boys. Should I slam on the brakes and scream out like a little girl? Maybe they would think we are about to be in an accident. Should I take them to one of the other schools in town and see if they recognize it or just find themselves standing there, watching me drive off into the darkness, wondering where their rides are. Finally, I decide. No, I'd better just take them to the high school where their parents are waiting.

As I turn off the highway and start over the bridge into the south part of town, I can see some of the boys waking up and wiping the sleep from their eyes. One asks, "What time is it?"

Looking at the time on the dash, I answer as I pull into the parking lot at the high school, "It's 2:00 a.m. and time for you guys to wake up and go home."

Colby and I both hop out and help the boys get their gear out of the back, and I make sure all the boys have rides home, not leaving any to walk or be stranded.

As the last parent waves and sends out a thank-you, Colby and I jump back into the Ram and start our drive out of town for the fifteen-minute ride home.

"How was the drive?" Colby asks.

Thinking about all that I had recalled on the way home, not only knowing I don't have enough time to cover it all, I say a simple, "It was okay, very quiet." As I smile at him.

As we approach our driveway, I can see that we have gotten some snow while we have been gone, and not wanting to fight any chances of getting stuck driving up our quarter-mile-long driveway, I reach down and pull the shift lever, putting the Dodge into four-wheel drive. As I'm plowing through the new snow approaching the house, and knowing Colby will be just walking into the house and going to bed, I ask him if he would leave his basketball uniform in the laundry room so I can throw it into the wash.

I don't even think the transmission is in park when he opens his door and starts out, trudges through the snow, and opens the front door of the house, letting the dogs out. They all run out to greet me, and I smile as they pay their respects. Or are they wondering if they will ever be fed this evening or, in this case, early morning?

After making sure they have all done their business and made yellow snow, we go back into the house and all enter the laundry room to find Colby's gym bag sitting in the laundry hamper. I shake my head, knowing he didn't take the time to empty it, just tossed the entire bag into the hamper and headed to bed.

After feeding the dogs, I open the gym bag to a very undesirable smell that even causes the dogs to take a break from eating and sniff the air. I think they want to pee on it. As I empty the content into the washer, I then decide to just toss in the smelly bag as well. I add a few other items, some soap, then start the washer and leave the room with it running and the dogs chowing down.

After a long late-night drive like that, I can't go right to bed. I crash on the sofa and flip on the TV, and as I am still recalling some of the events that came back to me tonight on my long, lonely drive, I once again think to myself, *Maybe I should write a book!* Then I think, *I wonder if anyone would believe it.*

ABOUT THE AUTHOR

RAISED BY HIS father, a county fire chief, the author spent most of his time around fire stations and, as soon as he was old enough, volunteered and started what was to be a lifelong career of helping others. EMT training, paramedic school, and eventually nursing school would give him the needed education to finally fulfill his goal of becoming a trauma flight nurse.

CPSIA information can be obtained
at www.ICGtesting.com
Printed in the USA
LVHW012244070121
675968LV00017B/291